PERIOD.
THE END

PERIOD
THE END

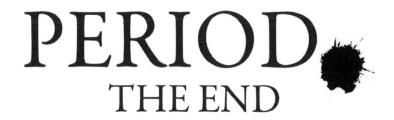

Wit, Wisdom, and Practical Guidance
for Women in Menopause–and Beyond

LINDA CONDRILLO

Cover design by Damonza
Interior design by Damonza
ISBN-13: 978-0-692-17936-9

For Kitten.

ACKNOWLEDGMENTS

This book would not be possible if not for the countless ladies who bravely came forth to share some of the least spoken—but most frequently wondered about—intimate details of their own menopausal life experiences, as well as the numerous medical experts and practitioners who contributed to this book. Thank you; you know who you are.

With warmest appreciation to Marlan K. Schwartz, MD, FACOG, FICS, who has seen more parts of my body than my own husband, for his expert advice from the day he told me I was pregnant with my daughter, through the trials and tribulations of my journey through menopause, and beyond.

To my long-suffering husband, Kent, who endured many of my menopausal meltdowns—and didn't run. To my children—Robert and Natalie, and Michael, my angel in heaven—who remind me never to take anything for granted, and that life is indeed a gift.

PROLOGUE

If she didn't know better, a woman entering menopause might think she woke up one day in a perpetual state of pregnancy, labor, and delivery. Menstruation ceases, her waistline nearly doubles, and undisturbed sleep soon becomes a thing of the past. The lucky who do reach the land of nod are awakened by cold sweats, bizarre dreams, and the need to pee, about every 20 minutes, in that order. Chocolate is officially classified as a new food group (and new drug of choice), often leading to what appears to be a permanent oversized muffin top. Sex, unexpectedly and suddenly, very often, becomes painfully impossible—either physically, mentally, or both.

Hot flashes arrive with as remarkable frequency as contractions during labor, except they don't completely disappear (in some cases) for a decade (or what seems like one). And instead of a little one trapped (temporarily) inside our body, *we* feel trapped inside our own bodies, try as we might to find some way, *any* way, to jump out of our own skin.

But whether or not you've been blessed with offspring, or never having experienced any part of childbirth by choice or by chance, giving birth to your menopausal self is inescapable.

When it's all over, there's no adorable package to coo over—just you, crying like a baby.

So, no surprise, some of the very same advice applicable throughout pregnancy is also relevant to making the most out of the next—and final—chapter of womanhood.

But hang on for the ride, ladies. Surviving *and thriving* menopause is possible—in fact, it's 100 percent conceivable!

CONTENTS

CONTENTS

By Angela DeRosa, M.D.

MENOPAUSE ... How does one word evoke so much fear in women and the population at large? It has been the topic of many stories, old wives' tales, books, and even musicals. One often wonders how our grand-mothers coped in silence!

Menopause is the "fat lady singing," but the retirement of the ovary is a slow and steady process, and for most of us, it can take more than a decade to get there. Women can have a whole host of symptoms prior to "period; the end." The more we talk about it out in the open, warts and all, the better we can care for ourselves and our fellow sisters in "hot flashes."

Period. The End is a humorous take on this serious topic while simultaneously providing sage advice for people who want a more holistic approach to dealing with the matter. If you want to ruminate less, sleep more, or find ways to brew teas and soothing baths, then you need to read this book.

As a menopause survivor, having gone through it at the young age of 35, I wish that I had some of these coping strategies. If a doctor says you are too young to have hormone deficiency, don't walk, *run*, out the door.

As a female internist and hormonal specialist, who is also nicknamed "Dr. Hot Flash," I have found a common warrior in Linda Condrillo as she gives women some much-needed information and coping strategies. I laughed, I cried, and I peed my pants a little when I read this book.

I have seen thousands of women over the past 28 years of practicing medicine and believe we all could use some laughter mixed in with our proverbial medicine. Hormone replacement therapy ultimately can treat the root cause of the many debilitating symptoms of hormone decline and menopause, and it should not be feared—despite what one may hear in the media. But for those who want additional options, or for women for whom hormone therapy is not appropriate, this book is just what the doctor ordered.

Dr. Angela DeRosa, also known as "Dr. Hot Flash," is an internal medicine doctor and a hormone and menopausal specialist at DeRosa Medical with offices in Scottsdale, Chandler, and Glendale, Arizona.

BIDDING ADIEU TO AUNT FLO

It seems like it was just yesterday I was a teenager in the '70s, preparing for dear Aunt Flo's very first arrival. Like many of her generation, my dear ol' Mum never revealed anything to me about "that time of the month" or what would happen when Aunt Flo finally did come to visit.

Instead, I'd learned what accommodations she'd need by memorizing every single word I read on the back of a box of sanitary napkins. What did "keep blue line away from body" mean anyway? For years, I wondered what would happen if the blue line actually *did* touch my body. Sadly, I couldn't even turn to my own mother for the answer.

But at the age of 16, getting my period was imminent, and after seeing the movie *Carrie,* I was determined to have a plan. If it weren't for my home economics teacher and a filmstrip she showed one afternoon, I might never have known what on earth a sanitary strap was put on this planet for, nor why I needed one to go with that big box of Kotex.

As the saying goes, "We've come a long way, baby!" Today's period protection is vastly better and easier to use than what my 16-year-old self had to use. But wouldn't you know it: Just about the time when they finally perfected a thin enough maxi to fit over a thong, I approached the age when I longer had any use for them—the maxi pads, anyway.

So, what's it like to lose your dear "friend," who has shown up like clockwork every 28th day since you were in the 10th grade, preempted only by an occasional self-imposed scare brought on by teenage ignorance or pregnancy or both—yikes.

Who knew that periods don't disappear as quickly as they once arrived? What's ahead? Long stretches of up to a year before they're gone for good—that's what. And that's just for starters. Because when menstruation stops, that's merely the beginning of menopause.

But wait, there's more! Mood swings, crying spells, and hot flashes, oh my! Now that I think about it, surely Carrie's mother must have been in full-blown menopause.

Alas, I suppose I should count my blessings, including my reproductive organs, which are thankfully still intact. Some of my friends have not been so lucky. But parting with dear Aunt Flo was bittersweet.

Ironically, my menopausal journey began just as my 12-year-old daughter was entering puberty. Careful not to make history repeat itself (or horrors, a sequel to *Carrie*), I was thrilled to pass the baton, along with every detail she wanted to know. We made plans to celebrate the day her period arrived, to go shopping together for thin maxis, perhaps even tampons, and giggle in the aisle past the adult diapers.

In the meantime, I'll chalk up my constant irritability and weight gain to menopause—and try not to blame my mother, God rest her soul.

Etymology: *Peri- 'around' + menopause*
Definition: *Pertaining to the time leading up to menopause when estrogen levels begin to drop*

CHAPTER 1

Are You Peri-Menopausal?

How do you know when you have officially started your journey into menopause? Is there a blood test? The answer is yes, of course there's a blood test—and great news—there aren't any needles involved! All you have to do is track your increasingly irregular periods. When they have stopped altogether for an entire year, you have officially arrived at the last stage of womanhood.

In the meantime, there are lots of ways to keep tabs on visits from Aunt Flo.

Free and interactive tools to help you *track your period* are available on the Internet here:

http://www.mymonthlycycles.com/perimenopause_tracker.jsp. Printable menstrual calendars are available online at: *http://www.menopause.org/docs/*

default-source/2015/menonote-menstrual-calendar-english.pdf. (You may want to print multiple copies.)

You can even find a variety of period tracking apps for mobile phones, which are detailed in this link from *Womens Health magazine*: *http://www.womenshealthmag.com/health/womanly-woes-theres-an-app-for-that.*

You might have also heard of home menopause testing kits, which measure the presence of follicle stimulating hormones (FSH) in the urine. What is FSH? It's a hormone produced by your pituitary gland. FSH levels increase temporarily each month to stimulate your ovaries to produce eggs. When you enter menopause and your ovaries stop working, your FSH levels also increase.

It's important to understand, however, tests results may be variable because during the time when periods are irregular, FSH levels can fluctuate widely. Women may have terrible menopause symptoms and yet their FSH level may remain in the pre- or perimenopausal range. Conversely, women without symptoms such as hot flashes still might have a FSH level in the menopausal range.

That's why the best thing to do when you suspect you're beginning to experience any sign of menopause is to see your health care provider.

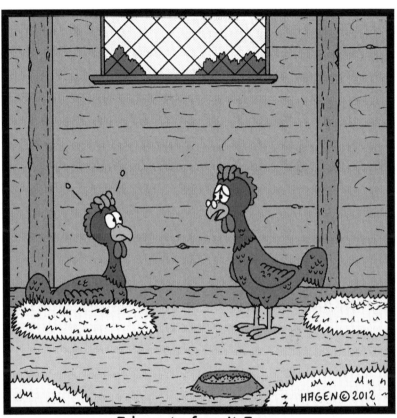

I have to face it Irma,
I haven't laid an egg in a week now: I'm menopausal...

Menopause: Signs, Symptoms, and Probable Causes

Sign	Symptom(s)	Probable Cause(s)
Absence of monthly period	Spotting, irregular periods, heavier flows	Lowered production of the female sex hormones estrogen and progesterone
Hot flashes	A sudden feeling of rising heat, usually starting in the upper portion of the body, face, and neck, or all over the body. Hot flashes can last anywhere from few seconds to several minutes, and they can occur at any time of the day or night.	Still a medical mystery
Insomnia	Changes in sleep patterns, difficulty falling or staying asleep, vivid dreams or nightmares, often exacerbated by night sweats	Hormone fluctuation
Urinary incontinence	Loss of control of bladder, frequent or painful urination	Loss of elasticity in vagina and urethra, weakening of surrounding pelvic muscles

Sign	Symptom(s)	Probable Cause(s)
Painful intercourse	Vaginal dryness and/or vaginal atrophy, bleeding during intercourse	Decreased production of estrogen and progesterone resulting in thinning vaginal walls
No interest in sex	Loss of libido, inability to climax	Vaginal dryness/ atrophy, feeling less desirable
Mood swings	Uncontrolled rage, mild to severe depression, irritability	Fluctuating hormones
Weight gain	Belly fat, muffin tops, the presence of a "second stomach"	Age-related inactivity, resulting in loss of muscle mass and lowered metabolism (Dropping estrogen levels may also cause the body to use starches and sugar less effectively, increasing fat storage around the middle.)

"
"I knew I was officially in menopause when I opened a mail-order catalog and saw a throw pillow that read: 'I'm out of estrogen, and I have a gun,' and laughed out loud."

—Haralee Weintraub

2

Positively Menopausal

I f all of the signs and symptoms in Chapter One apply to you, congratulations! You're certifiably menopausal. You may be wondering, "When is this going to be over?" The truth is, every woman's journey from peri- to post-menopause is different. For some, it seems like forever, with many of us experiencing symptoms for up to a decade. Still others breeze through menopause with nary a hot flash.

According to Marlan Schwartz, MD, past chairman of the department of obstetrics and gynecology at Robert Wood Johnson University Hospital, in Somerset, New Jersey, the average age most women begin to enter menopause is approximately 51½ years.

To add insult to injury, many women can enter into menopause prematurely. Cancer-fighting drugs such as Tamoxifen have been known to induce menopausal symptoms. Surgical menopause results from the removal of both ovaries, and radiation and chemo-therapy can cause the ovaries to no longer function.

Menopause: "The New Hot"

Fans down, hot flashes, which are also called hot flushes, are the number one symptom most ladies have in common. Clinically known as vasomotor symptoms, hot flashes take most women by surprise. In fact, not everyone immediately recognizes a hot flash for what it is. It's sort of like the first time your baby kicks inside your womb. You're not really sure if it's the miracle of life—or gas.

Marianne J., just 44 at the time of her first hot flash, remembers it this way:

"I woke up in the middle of the night, dripping with sweat. I felt fine otherwise. The only reasonable explanation I could think of was that sometime while I was asleep, I must have run a fever, and by the time I woke up, it broke!"

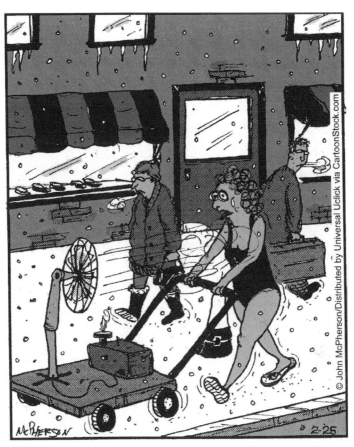

Kathy's hot flashes were becoming severe.

Here are some other firsthand descriptions from women well acquainted with hot flashes:

It felt as if someone literally took a blowtorch to me.

I would blow-dry my hair, and when I had finished, it was all wet again. I ended up sitting in front of the fan for 10 minutes to cool down before I would dry my hair for a second time.

It feels like someone turned up the heat, and then you look around and see you're the only one who feels it.

All night long, it's covers on, covers off, covers on, covers off. My poor little dog won't sleep with me anymore. She's tired of me flinging her against the wall.

You suddenly feel hot and sweaty and feel the need to tear off your clothes.

One minute you seem fine, and the next, you're trapped in a room full of heat with no escape.

It's like wearing a snowsuit with layers of cashmere undergarments while running on a treadmill inside a sauna.

This was the cycle: The nude run and then diving under a blanket, like a cold little kitten.

There are times I'll be walking in the winter and have to open my coat wide open to be able to breathe. I'll be sweating in 35-degree weather. It's crazy.

I like to keep my bedroom at meat-locker temperatures at night. I tossed and turned all last night just sweating. Was it the beer? The hibachi? Did I have a fever? Finally crawled out of bed a little after 6 to find the heat at 68. Someone turned the heat up at bedtime. Someone's gonna pay for that. And it's not gonna be pretty.

Menopausal Anomalies

Some women don't experience menopausal symptoms, or if they do, they don't attribute them to menopause.

"I may have had a hot flash in the early months," says Susan M., age 57. "It was more of a rush of warmth. I had a few of them, but they never really took hold. And then they stopped. Once in a rare while, I would wake up warm in the middle of the night, but I was always able to fall back to sleep.

"My periods were so regular. They resumed 28 days to the day after the birth of my first child, and 30 days after the birth of my second. I almost never suffered from cramps, and throughout my menstrual life, I never really thought about the whole process.

"So the time came, and my periods slowed. Each year, I would go to the doctor, and she would ask, 'So, how was the year?' I would say 'Okay.' She would ask if I had a period. Most of the time I said, 'I *think* so.' So she would say, 'Not done yet!' A few years into this routine, she said, 'You are done and now in meno-pause.' I said, 'Okay.' And that was that. I never gave it another thought. I have no fun stories, no events that have changed my thinking, and no impact to my life because of this non-event."

Susan simply attributes her attitude to working full-time and not really thinking about her body.

"I eat well. I sleep well. I have sex," Susan says. "I have no pains, no aches, and no physical issues. I keep my mind busy, and I am in constant motion. I like to travel, and I plan, plan, plan."

Mary H., age 80, felt helpless when her own daughter entered menopause in a very different way than she had. "I had no symptoms whatsoever. When I had my period, there was never any warning signs nor discomfort, not even a cramp. One day I got it, and then, when I was about 50, one day it just stopped. I feel terrible that I can't answer any questions or relate to what my daughter is going through."

Menopause "was a breeze" for Laurie T., age 56, who also enjoyed an uneventful change.

"I thought the fear-mongering was ridiculous," Laurie says. "We women were supposed to be afraid, very afraid of menopause. It was a sign that we were aging! (As if men don't age!) Our skin was going to get wrinkly! (As if men don't wrinkle.) I had a hard time taking all the hype seriously. It was a liberation."

Laurie attributes her ease into and quick exit out of menopause to observing a purely plant-based (vegan) diet.

Blair S., age 60, was also spared most menopausal complaints. "I really only got the hot flashes, which I viewed as going through the transition to the next stage of my life. When I experienced one, it felt like being in Florida (especially in the cooler months), so I would refer to those hot flashes as 'my own personal Florida.' I think saying that to myself would give me an image of palm trees, blue skies, gentle waves on the Gulf or ocean, and lying on the beach with a vodka tonic! And quite frankly it was a gift to get my mind somewhere else, especially during difficult days! I also feel like I'm 18—until I look in the mirror, that is! I don't want to stop and think about any age-related issues. And my grandchildren definitely keep me young!"

Too Soon, Too Soon!

Dana R. can't swear her meltdowns were attributed to menopause entirely. She says menopause "took a backseat" when she lost her husband when she was just 47.

"I didn't know what hit me ... Right after Jim died, I had so many emotional lows, it was impossible to tell if I was in full-blown menopause or just suffering in general with the loss of my husband, trying to cope, with moderate bouts of depression."

Left with two school-age children, Dana says she "was in a fog for about three years."

Jennifer R. was just 44 when she got a "fast pass to menopause." A series of abnormal Pap smears led to the ultimate recommendation to have a hysterectomy. "Although my ovaries were not removed, they were fried by eight weeks of radiation. Yet, I came through it all stronger and better than ever, and I don't miss having my period one bit."

At the age of 38, Gai C. was diagnosed with breast cancer. "I didn't enter the dreaded zone naturally. Tamoxifen almost immediately stopped my periods. I was 'forced' into menopause. Doctors say that medically induced menopause is more intense. Hot flashes were like rushes up my neck and head in the beginning. Sometimes my chest would go on fire. I never had time to dwell on the 'changes' or on feeling out of sorts. I was in the throes of months of radiation treatments, every day. I had every symptom from hot and cold sweats all day, every day, for years; mood swings bordering on depression, night sweats, sleeplessness … and if that wasn't enough, I was bald.

"I remember the first time I noticed goose flesh on my arms but I was not registering cold. With my chemo treatments, I lost all of my hair. Because the hot flashes were intense on my face, I found myself more than once with a drawn-on eyebrow heading south down my face.

"But when you're with a group of the same women in a hospital out-patient radiology office, believe me, you don't talk about your flashes. You talk vacation, sales at the mall, the kids, etc., anything but medical crap. It was much harder and much longer as the chemo and Tamoxifen intensified and prolonged the symptoms. The interesting thing for me [being so young] was that friends my own age weren't experiencing the same things. I ended up seeking solace with a group of ladies from our car club, who were much older and going through menopause. They were a Godsend."

Another breast cancer survivor, Joy K., reminds us to count our blessings. "We have to be oh so thankful for going through menopause. I know some women who never had the chance."

Don't Panic, It's Only an Anxiety Attack; It'll be Over, Right After the Hot Flash!

Changes in your heart rate are common right before or during a hot flash. It may become rapid, or irregular, and you may feel heart palpitations. So it's hard to tell which comes first: the panic attack or the hot flash.

"When the adrenals are no longer protected by sufficient magnesium, the fight-or-flight hormones, adrenaline and noradrenaline, become more easily triggered," says Carolyn Dean, MD, ND, a medical advisory board member of the Nutritional Magnesium Association at www.nutritionalmagnesium.org. "When they surge erratically, they cause a rapid pulse, high blood pressure, and heart palpitations. The more magnesium-deficient you are, the more exaggerated is the adrenaline response. Magnesium calms the nervous system, relaxes muscle tension, and lowers the pulse rate, helping to reduce anxiety and panic attacks."

Dr. Dean says it's "absolutely important" for menopausal women to take a magnesium supplement. She adds, "According to the USDA, 100 years ago we were getting 500 mg per day of magnesium; now we're lucky to get 200 mg." Dr. Dean believes the average person needs 600 mg, not the 350mg that is the current RDA. Dr. Dean also notes, "Not all forms of magnesium are easily absorbed by the body. Magnesium citrate powder is a highly absorbable form that can be mixed in hot or cold water and sipped throughout the day." Your doctor can order a blood test to determine whether or not you are deficient in magnesium.

Dr. Angela DeRosa, an internal medicine doctor and a hormone and menopausal specialist adds, "Magnesium and adrenal balancing are very important to better manage our stress levels, but even more importantly, if we are deficient in testosterone, we lack proper serotonin firing in the brain. Our reactions to stress are magnified, and we lose our ability to cope."

Roxanne R., age 53, says her hot flashes seem to come in waves, and they are brought on many times by anxiety. "Sometimes they come at the most inopportune times, including when I'm meeting with clients, many of whom are men. I break out in a noticeable sweat, which is so embarrassing that I have to excuse myself to go to the bathroom."

Moms entering menopause right at the time when their children are learning how to drive a car or preparing to leave home to go to college or live on their own are particularly prone to added stress over the "what ifs."

"I'd drift off, in and out of sleep on the couch in front of the TV, waiting for my daughter to come in, or to get a text to let me know she was on her way, and I'd wake up in an absolute panic, my heart pounding out of my chest, my clothes soaked with sweat, not knowing if I'd heard the door close or if I was dreaming," says Grace C., age 59. "All kinds of worry go through your mind. If the curfew is 10 p.m. and the kid isn't in the house by 10:01, you worry. At 10:05, you worry more. If she's not home by 10:10, you're panicked and now want to call or text to see where she is, but you have to stop yourself because you don't want to call or text if she is actually in the car driving, because you don't want her to use the phone while she's driving. So you wait it out. When you can't stand it any longer, you call, but then get the recording you get when the phone is off. Or the text comes back as undeliverable. You pace around the house, imagining any and every "worst case" scenario. Finally she walks in the door, and you turn into *your* mother."

If you've convinced yourself that your kids are all right, you move on to worrying about your parents. 56-year-old Donna R.'s husband, Mark, summed up his wife's logic this way: "If she calls her mother and the phone rings and rings and she doesn't pick up, there's only one possible explanation: She's dead."

Some women joke the proper terminology for the change of life should be changed to "mental-pause." Keeping a sense of humor does help, along with taking numerous deep cleansing breathes and remembering "this too shall pass."

Joy G., 56, finds taking a regular yoga class helps calm her anxiety, at least temporarily. "I'm finding exercise and meditation to help a great deal, and yoga is a little bit of both."

Lynette Sheppard, the author of *Becoming a Menopause Goddess* and webmistress of the *Menopausal Goddess blog*, describes the correlation between menopause and anxiety this way: "Nighttime anxiety takes on a distressing theme of instant replays. Like a curmudgeonly version of the movie *Groundhog Day*, you're forced to relive over and over some insignificant event. Ordinary moments play over and over in your brain like visual earworms. You review the dinner where you had an extra glass of wine and told an overlong story about your cats. You see yourself over and over again saying something stupid to your neighbor. A little episode of mutual crankiness at the dinner table plays *ad nauseam*. Even a mundane phone conversation with your mother is stuck on repeat.

"Yet unlike that uplifting movie where Bill Murray learns the meaning of life and love, you just keep viewing the same loop with no resolution in sight. You know that in the morning it will strike you as inconsequential and meaningless, even silly, but right now in the dark of night, it won't leave you alone."

Lynette recommends repeating what she calls the menopausal mantra: "This too shall pass. This is a natural process, and with a little help from your friends, you *will* be able to find your balance once again."

Over-the-counter herbs, such as black cohosh, may provide some relief from hot flashes. Homeopathic remedies, such as cinnamon, ashwagandha, licorice, and shatavari, also might help.

Patricia N. experienced "a dramatic turnaround" after taking *Dr. Tobias's Women Hormonal Balance & Menopause Support Capsules*. She says, "I do still experience a teeny bit of a flash every now and again—maybe once a day. I won't even notice until I walk past a mirror and see just a tiny bit of dewiness around my hairline. It's finger-snap quick, not the miserable drawn-out sessions they used to be."

Mindfulness matters. Many women seek solace in prayer, meditation, and taking time out to simply breathe.

Communing with nature (or playing recorded nature sounds on CD), adopting a diet of "clean" (whole, unprocessed), foods, as well as keeping regularly scheduled visits to the gym, chiropractor, acupuncturist, masseuse, or manicurist may also help the typical day in a menopausal woman's life.

"I walk my dog half a mile, three times a day," says Rhonda F., age 59, "It gives me a chance to 'get out of my head' at least for a while, and I'm mindful that she won't be around for more than a few more years. I try to appreciate these moments with the dog, savor them actually, as ordinary as they may be, and try to create as many happy moments I can throughout the day."

Always remember to consult a physician before starting any new diet, supplement, or exercise regimens.

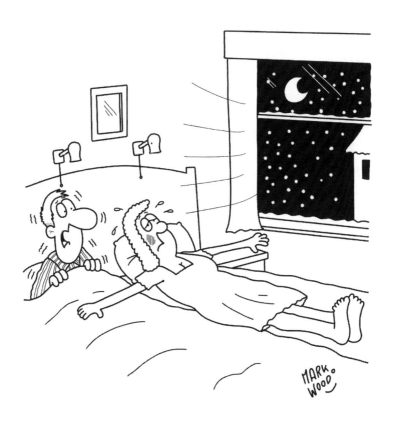

"H..has your hot flush gone yet? C..can
we close the window now?"

CHAPTER 3

SOS (Save Our Sleep)

Sleep, Sweat, Repeat

Because hot flashes often occur in the evening hours, getting a good night's rest seems next to impossible for budding menopausal insomniacs.

Once Mr. Sandman finally arrives, many women awake abruptly, dripping in sweat. Sheets and pajamas are often soaked through and need to be changed, sometimes more than once each night.

Environmental sleep specialist Anita Mahaffey attributes night sweats as one of the primary reasons for starting her company, *Cool-jams, Inc.* Mahaffey's company developed cooling pillows and covers, blankets, sheets, and sleepwear to help the restless achieve the optimum sleep temperature range.

According to Mahaffey, "Researchers have shown that insomniacs tend to have warmer core body temperatures than normal sleepers just before bed, which leads to heightened arousal and a struggle to fall asleep. For troubled sleepers, a cool room and a hot-water bottle placed at the feet, which rapidly dilates blood vessels and therefore actually helps lower core body temperature, can push the internal thermostat to a better setting."

Thrown into menopause by chemotherapy, breast cancer survivor Haralee Weintraub's hot flashes were off the charts. "I went from someone being cold all the time to someone sweating all the time."

A true champion for the cause, Weintraub started a specialty garment business to help other women achieve relief from night sweats and other menopausal side effects. *Haralee.com*'s "Cool Garments for Hot Women" are beautifully designed pajamas made of moisture-wicking polyester with sweat-transporting fibers that are breathable and fast drying. Weintraub donates a percentage of the profits to breast cancer research.

Sleep in a Bottle

Waking up several times during the night and trying to fall back to sleep becomes a vicious cycle. At one point, Weintraub turned to her doctor for a prescription remedy, which provided a temporary fix.

"I could not turn off my brain. I tried all the drugs, but the one that worked best for me was Lunesta (3 milligrams). Personally, I had no side effects from the drug. I went off it because I noticed I was able to fall asleep on my own again, and when I wake up, I can usually fall back to sleep."

Lauren B., age 58, also went the Rx route. "There was a time in my own life when I 'couldn't live' without Ambien," she recalls. "I was commuting to New York at the time, leaving my house by 7 a.m., and frequently putting in 12-hour days. I was too wound up to fall asleep on my own, and when I did, I would wake up a few hours later and would remain that way until about 5 a.m., when I'd finally drift off asleep about 45 minutes before my alarm went off.

"Falling asleep and staying asleep seemed impossible without the drug, and my family was worried about the possibility of me being 'hooked.' Even if it was the weekend, or I was on vacation, I felt psychologically dependent upon it, which is when I began to worry myself. I gradually weaned myself off, eventually stopped taking it completely, and am now finally able to fall asleep and stay asleep for a stretch of about six hours. Not perfect, but I'll take it. Plus, I still have a stash, just in case I need it."

Because not much is known about long-term sleep medication use, most of them are recommended only for short periods of time and used with caution, including over-the-counter sleep aids.

Carolyn Dean, MD, ND, a medical advisory board member of the Nutritional Magnesium Association at www.nutritionalmagnesium.org, says that magnesium deficiency has been strongly linked to sleep disorders, which can either cause or increase anxiety. "If you're stressed out, not sleeping, tense, and irritable, taking a good magnesium supplement could pull you out of that downward spiral."

Another category of natural sleep remedies available without a prescription and growing in popularity are essential oils. Proponents suggest lavender oil (*Lavandula angustifolia*), for example, may help promote a restful night's sleep.

But not all essential oils are created equal, as many are not safe for topical use and are intended for aromatherapy only.

Orest Pelechaty, LAc, OMD, a doctor of Oriental Medicine who is nationally certified in acupuncture and Chinese herbal medicine and the clinic director at the *Center for Integrated Holistic Medicine* in Springfield, New Jersey, warns, "Most essential oils on the market should be avoided like the plague." He advises people seek out *only* essential oils that are held to the strictest of standards from seed to seal. According to Dr. Pelechaty, the Young Living brand is one of the leaders in terms of purity. (Their products can be ordered online from www.YoungLiving.com.) "Lavender in particular is very good for anxiety, as it resolves tension and is very grounding."

Filling a glass pump bottle with distilled water, and adding several drops of lavender oil to spritz your pillow before bedtime may ensure a good night's rest. Or enjoy a cool mist aromatherapy experience by adding several drops of lavender essential oil to a cold water diffuser.

Doris Harrison, a distributor for Young Living Essential Oils, shares this recipe for a relaxing bath salt, sure to create a relaxing nighttime ritual.

> **Note:** For any essential oil recipes involving bath or massage blends, be sure to choose an essential oil labeled safe for topical use. Always dilute the essential oil with a carrier oil and test on a small part of your skin for sensitivity before using. If there is skin sensitivity, apply a carrier oil (such as olive or coconut) to the affected area and wipe off. Or wipe the area dry, apply soap directly to a washcloth, completely work the soap into the area first without water, and then rinse off.

Doris's Relaxing Blend

What You'll Need:

- Mixing bowl
- Spoon
- Storage container, such as a glass jar, if you're multiplying the recipe to make more than you'll need for 1 bath
- Label
- Decorative embellishments (optional)
- Unscented candles for ambience (optional)

1 cup Epsom salt (pure magnesium flakes)

½ cup baking soda (optional)

5 drops Young Living Release essential oil blend

4 drops Young Living Geranium essential oil

3 drops Young Living Patchouli essential oil

2 drops Young Living Lavender essential oil

How to Make It:

In the bowl, mix the salt, baking soda (if desired), and Young Living essential oils. Gently stir with the spoon. When mixed well, transfer the bath salts to the jar. Label and decorate the jar if desired.

As you prepare your bath, close the bathroom window and door to prevent oil vapors from escaping. Fill the bathtub with warm/not-too-hot water so the oils don't vaporize before you can take advantage of the benefits.

Because essential oils evaporate quickly, dissolve 1 cup of the mixture in the bathwater just prior to bath time. With your hand, swirl the water to disperse the mixture evenly, then carefully enter the bath. Arrange candles in desired location and relax and enjoy the bath for at least 30 minutes.

Exotic Floral Bath Salts

What You'll Need:

- Mixing bowl
- Spoon
- Storage container, such as a glass jar, if you're multiplying the recipe to make more than you'll need for 1 bath
- Label
- Decorative embellishments (optional)
- Unscented candles (optional)
- 1 cup Epsom salt or dead sea salt
- 5 drops Young Living Jasmine essential oil
- 5 drops Young Living Ylang Ylang essential oil

How to Make It:

In the bowl, mix the salt and Young Living essential oils. Gently stir with the spoon. When mixed well, transfer the bath salts to the jar. Label and decorate the jar if desired.

As you prepare your bath, close the bathroom window and door to prevent oil vapors from escaping. Fill the bathtub with warm/not-too-hot water so the oils don't vaporize before you can take advantage of the benefits.

Because essential oils evaporate quickly, dissolve 1 cup of the mixture in the bathwater just prior to bath time. With your hand, swirl the water to disperse the mixture evenly, then carefully enter the bath. Place the candles in desired location and relax and enjoy the bath for at least 30 minutes.

Caution should always be used when using essential oils, and Harrison advises avoiding any spicy, minty, or "hot" oils in the bath. Some examples are peppermint, wintergreen, basil, oregano, thyme, black pepper, or bay leaf oils, all of which could cause irritation, especially on sensitive skin.

After enjoying a relaxing bath, you might savor a warm drink just before bedtime.

Holistic Health Coach *Sarah Lawrence* suggests a delicious turmeric-infused coconut milk elixir to improve digestion, calm the nervous system, and prepare for restful sleep. You'll see the best results over time as the ingredients in the elixir work to repair and replenish your body.

Lawrence shares this delicious recipe from her article in *www.fitlife.tv*

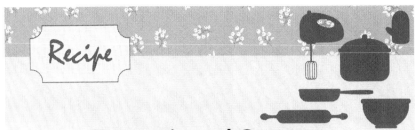

Turmeric and Coconut Milk Bedtime Elixir

What You'll Need:

Serves: 4

- 4 cups coconut milk

- 2 tsp powdered turmeric or 2 tbsp peeled, fresh turmeric

- 2 tsp powdered ginger or 2 tbsp peeled, fresh ginger

- ¼ tsp ground nutmeg

- 1 tbsp coconut oil

- 2 tbsp maple syrup, raw honey, or a squirt of liquid stevia

- 12 peppercorns, gently crushed

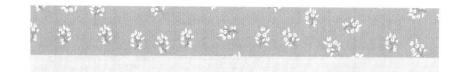

How to Make It:

Combine everything except the coconut oil and sweetener in a saucepan and bring to a simmer.

Let the mixture bubble gently for about 5 minutes, then shut off the heat.

After about 5 minutes of cooling, strain the mixture through a few layers of cheesecloth or a very fine strainer if you prefer a smoother texture.

Stir in the coconut oil.

Taste and add maple syrup, honey or stevia if desired.

Cry Uncle

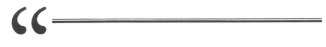

*I haven't slept through the
night in like, forever.*

—*Jeri G., 58*

Social media support groups for menopausal women are plentiful and are open 24/7. Facebook posts are commonplace in the menopausal world in the wee hours of the night.

Nutritional therapist and natural menopause practitioner Vikki Ede started a Facebook page called *Menopause Support Group* to raise awareness after suffering (and ultimately resolving) her own "perimenopausal nightmare."

By her own admission, Vikki is a "hormone geek," who loves giving women ages 40 and older the tools to "take charge of the change." Her mission is to shake up menopause, get everyone talking about it, help women stop suffering the debilitating symptoms, and eradicate the social taboo. Within the Menopause Support Group Facebook page, Vikki shares her advice, including simple natural solutions to find hormonal health and happiness with fellow members.

"I created the Menopause Support Group Facebook page to be a space where women could ask all those crazy questions going around in their heads and to let them know that they are not alone."

With thousands of members from around the globe, someone's always up and ready to lend a supportive ear and offer advice on whatever's ailing a member.

Join the Menopause Support Group Facebook page here:

*https://www.facebook.com/groups/
AllThingsMenopauseSupportGroup*
or visit
http://menopausesupportgroup.com.

If you find you *still* can't sleep, venturing out of the bedroom and into a quiet place to read can help. Some menopausal women find 3 in the morning just as good a time as any to clean their bathrooms, do other work around the house, or spend some quality time online.

"I've done my floors, three loads of laundry, and changed the cat litter at 3:45 on many an occasion."— Kimberly T.

"There were years of sleepless nights for me. I'd wake up around 2 a.m. and not be able to fall back asleep. Finally, I just gave up and got out of bed and painted my entire kitchen!"—Dana W.

Lynette Sheppard calls this special part of a day in the life of menopausal women the "night of the undones."

"[Once in bed], you remain awake, thinking of those things you forgot to do, should have done, or worry that you might need to do," Sheppard says. "It's like thought zombies that parade through your night, jostling you, keeping you awake with silent incessant nagging. Did I pay last month's phone bill? I can't remember seeing it. I forgot to call the plumber or clean the cat box. I should have bought computer paper. When did I last check the oil in the car? What am I going to do with all those Christmas cards I bought, now that it is mid-January? Did I buy laundry soap? Did I clean the lint catcher in the dryer? The litany goes on. And on.

"If I got up and wrote these little reminders down, I'd be up for a while. Usually, I would stay in bed, trying to focus enough to commit them to memory in case they might be important. However, this took long enough that I'd be up anyway. If I tried to ignore the undone zombies, they just kept lurching into my consciousness, and I'd be up. Forget about using one of those little light pens that you can use to write down your list in the middle of the night, guaranteed to keep you from waking your spouse and to allow you to fall right back to sleep, safe in the knowledge that you have corralled and organized the zombies. Suffice it to say that I'd fumble around in the dark, knocking all other implements from my bedside table to the floor, searching for this small item that, if I weren't so irritated, would help me so much. But then, I'd be frustrated and heading toward pissed off, so once again I was awake and up for a while. The only thing that seemed to help dissipate the night-time anxiety was anger.

"The one thing that truly made it all bearable was knowing that I was not the only one. I knew my menopausal sisters were there—in some other car, riding along with me, sharing my sweats and terrors. And knowing that this was normal. And temporary."

Sleep? Dream On (Crazy Dreams)

Once menopausal women finally fall asleep, they are often plagued by wild and crazy dreams. This is another way menopause mirrors pregnancy. Dreams during menopause can often be very intense—vivid and scary. Perhaps this is completely normal, considering the amount of anxiety experienced during menopause—and aging in general.

"My dreams seem like hours-long feature films, vivid and detailed in full color and ranges of emotions," says Kathleen S., age 63, an author, ghostwriter, and presenter from Olympia, Washington.

Kathleen says she "practically lives" on sites like *Dream Dictionary* because "part of me wonders if I could figure out what the heck is bothering me, maybe the dreams wouldn't be so intense. I'll wake up exhausted from some of them, drained, because I've been angry or frustrated during the dream.

"I've always been a dreamer, but menopause stirs the hormonal pot, the dredges of what's left of hormones in our bodies," she adds. "I think the dreams get more intense at times, sort of like hot flashes in your sleep."

Many menopausal women experience reoccurring dreams of being lost, waking up in a sweat or even shaking. Other reoccurring dreams for many are being naked or hiding where no one can see them.

Why do menopausal women have these vivid dreams? An article published in *More* magazine by Kristal Brent Zook, *"How Your Dreams Change over Decades,"* suggests there may be a connection between midlife hormonal changes and sleep.

The article states that research has shown that depression and insomnia, two conditions that often become more frequent during the menopausal transition, are known to speed up the production of rapid eye movements (REMs), which occur during the stage most closely associated with dreams.

"Generally speaking, if you have more intense REM periods, there will be more activity and emotionality in your dreams," says Joseph De Koninck, PhD, director of the sleep laboratory at the University of Ottawa, Ontario.

Stretch and Breathe

The *National Sleep Foundation* recommends practicing the following exercise as you lie down to go to sleep, and also if you wake up during the night and have trouble falling back to sleep. This is especially helpful if you find your mind racing or preoccupied with too many thoughts to allow you to drift off to sleep. The idea is to continue to redirect your attention to your breathing and your body anytime you find yourself lost in thought. When you let thoughts go and simply keep your attention on your breathing, you are better able to welcome sleep.

Find a comfortable position in bed. Let yourself relax and start to notice your body and any sensations you feel. Feel the connection between your body and the surface you're lying on. Relax any tension and soften your muscles.

Focus your attention on your body. If your mind starts to wander to thoughts or worries, gently bring it back to your body. It's very common to become preoccupied while you're lying in bed. It takes time and practice to learn how to focus your attention on the body only. Start to notice your breath and where you feel it in your body. You might feel it in your abdomen, your chest, or your nostrils. Focus your attention on the full breath, from start to finish. If your mind is wandering, just notice that it has wandered and gently redirect it back to your breath.

Take a deep breath into your lower belly (not your chest) and feel your abdomen expand with air. Hold this for a few seconds and then release. Notice your belly rising and falling, and the air coming in and out a few times. Imagine the air filling up your abdomen and then traveling out your airways, over and over.

Continue to do this for a few minutes, focusing your mind on your body and the breath coming in and out. Anytime a thought crosses your mind, release that thought and refocus on your breath. Feel yourself relaxing even more deeply. Practice this silently for a few minutes.

Do a scan of your body while you lie down, noticing anywhere you might feel tension. Review the areas of your body, starting from the top of your head and moving all the way to your toes, relaxing the tension when you encounter it. As you do this, direct your breath into that area of your body to help you release that tension.

After you have scanned your body, return to the simple breathing pattern, continuing to notice your breath and picturing it flowing into and out of your belly.

Attack of the Charley Horse

Even if menopausal women have no issues with sleep—or the lavender oil kicks in and they finally drift off to dreamland—many women awake with excruciating leg pain, usually in the calf muscle. This type of pain is generally referred to as a "charley horse."

With as many hours as we spend sitting at the computer for work or for play, it comes as no surprise that this sort of inactivity may be the cause of a leg cramp, or even a "dead leg." We get up, walk around, the pain and pins and needles subside, and we return to "normal."

"Charley horse" is just another name for a muscle spasm. Charley horses can occur in virtually any muscle, but they are most common in the legs. These spasms are marked by extremely uncomfortable muscle contractions. The muscles don't relax for several seconds or more, and the pain can be quite severe.

Although charley horses are common at night, they can also occur when you're awake, relaxing on the sofa, or even standing up.

"Once you're in [charley horses], they don't have an off switch!" says Kathy S., who calls herself the "cramp queen." "I've tried quinine, drinking more water and even vinegar, and eating bananas, but the problem is I forget and then suffer [cramps in my] calf muscles or my feet (ankles and toes) miserably. Then I'm good about trying to remember to take care of myself. But isn't that a twofold issue because we don't remember things well and the leg cramps hurt like hell."

Charley horses are generally treatable at home, especially if they are infrequent. If they are persistent, it's best to check with your doctor and ask for help in determining the cause, as well as implementing treatments and preventive measures to increase your comfort.

A number of factors may cause a *muscle to cramp* or spasm. One of the most common causes of charley horses is inadequate blood flow to the muscle, which is called blood vacuity. Too little calcium, potassium, or sodium in the blood may also play a role.

Eating nutrient-dense foods, especially those rich in phosphorous, magnesium, and potassium, whenever possible may reduce the frequency of leg cramps. Foods such as cheese, yogurt, nuts and seeds, legumes, grains such as quinoa, and brown rice, as well as avocados, oranges, salmon, turkey, and chicken are excellent sources.

"Magnesium is intimately involved in efficient muscle function," says Carolyn Dean, MD, ND, author of *The Magnesium Miracle*. "The mechanisms are varied and include oxygen uptake, electrolyte balance, and energy production. Magnesium makes muscles work properly, allowing calcium to cause muscle contraction and then pushing calcium out of the muscle cells to allow the relaxation phase. In the same way that nerve cells can be 'excited to death,' muscle cells stimulated by too much calcium can go into uncontrollable spasm, resulting in tissue damage such as occurs in a heart attack.

"All muscles, including the heart and smooth muscles lining the blood vessels, contain more magnesium than calcium. If magnesium is deficient, calcium floods into the smooth muscle cells of blood vessels and causes spasms leading to constricted blood vessels and therefore higher blood pressure, arterial spasm, angina, and heart attack.[1] A proper balance of magnesium in relation to calcium can prevent these symptoms."

---

1   Teo KK et al., "Effects of intravenous magnesium in suspected acute myocardial infarction: overview of randomized trials." Brit Med J, vol. 303, pp. 1499–1503, 1991.

"

There are few things worse than perky, upbeat proclamations about how this is the best time of our lives. Eventually it may be, but we go through a few ridiculous years before we come out of the other side feeling whole again. Different, but whole. Menopause. It will set you free, but it will really mess with you first.

—Lynette Sheppard

CHAPTER 4

You're So Sensitive!

Things That Bug Me

Hyper awareness and/or hypersensitivity to odors and noises, including the sound of someone's annoying voice, is another common irritant menopausal women share. Whining children in restaurants, secondhand smoke that we hardly noticed in our younger days, and music spilling out of headphones from the person sitting next to us on a bus or train can send us into a rage. The ensuing complaining about it all can be equally irritating to our family and non-menopausal friends. However, it does make for some really funny Facebook rants.

Realizing the true meaning behind "life is short," we lack patience in listening to the mundane.

As it turns out, lack of patience seems to be a very common thread (who knew?), as these ladies have shared some common annoyances:

- *People who don't answer emails. A simple 'I'll get that to you by x' doesn't take long to type. And it keeps me from sending you repeated reminders, thinking that you didn't see my previous 87 emails.*

- *I find myself less nurturing and not really interested in the minutia of people's lives.*

- *The post office: Every time I go to mail a bill or send a package, do I really have to answer the same question over and over: 'Is this liquid, fragile, hazardous?' I'm tired of hearing all the 'options' I have. I just need a 48-cent stamp!*

- *The constant ping sound of texts going off non-stop on cell phones.*

- *The mere sight of a skinny Santa Claus, seriously!*

- *Lip smacking, gum chewing, or someone munching on popcorn, including the rustling of the bag at the movies!*

- *Ignorance from 'experts,' setting up (and being dependent upon) new electronic devices, nit-picking, waiting for almost anything, requests from people who feel entitled and forget to say thank you, and presumption of any kind without verbalization.*

- *In three words: Filling out forms!*

- *The clear rubbery straps on the inside of a shirt or dress, I just want to cut them off the minute I take the tags off!*

- *Teleprompters! I push '0' over and over, until I reach a live human being!*

- *Women who report 'I just breezed through menopause.' Or 'I never had any side effects with menopause because I work out so much and I am so fit.' … You know, 'superior attitude' women!*

Meltdowns, Irritability, and Mourning The Loss of Whatever Patience You Thought You Had Left

"I have always heard of women who become nuts once they become menopausal, but that has not been my issue—although my husband of 41 years may think differently."

—Carol Gee,
Author of Random Notes: About Life,
"Stuff" and Finally Learning to Exhale

Meltdowns and crying spells are commonplace in the menopausal world. Just about anything can set you off—a TV commercial, the sight of a dead cat on the side of the road, a scrapbook with homemade Mother's Day cards from your children. Don't be surprised if part of your daily routine includes tucking a tissue inside your sleeve.

"Crying seemed to be my outlet rather than screaming or ranting," says Gai C. "I pretty much cried whenever I was alone. I particularly seemed to like crying [on my drive] to and from work. From the time I pulled out of the garage at home until the time I got to work, I cried and didn't really seem to mind until people in the other cars gave me funny looks. Then the same thing on the way home. It was probably quite liberating as I have never been much of a crier."

"I've definitely had the 'sads' and the 'mads' more frequently," adds Roxanne R. "With the sads, I can, at times, cry uncontrollably even though nothing's really wrong. It's embarrassing when you're at a party and you have to go hide until this subsides and your eyes look like you've gone 10 rounds with melancholy."

Preserving your sense of humor can definitely help combat the bouts of despondency. "Menopause can really be a bitch for some of us ladies, while others are super fortunate to not experience a thing, not one hot flash," Roxanne continues. "But for those of you who have had to excuse yourself from a business meeting because you're dripping with sweat, have suddenly developed a pooch in the stomach area, have uncharacteristic mood swings or melancholy, let's commiserate, support each other, and try to have the last laugh."

This inspired Roxanne to write a song entitled "*Menopause Done Me Wrong.*" Find it on YouTube here:

https://www.youtube.com/watch?v=3N_auM2J05c.

Menopause Done Me Wrong

By Roxanne Rubell

First Verse

Menopause done me wrong

I can't fit in my thong

My jeans are tight

I can't sleep at night

I'm sweaty and bitchy

Oh what a sight

Menopause done me wrong

It started last year.

When Aunt Ruby disappeared.

She said goodbye

Now all I do is cry

Will I be this hot 'til the day I die?

Menopause done me wrong

Bridge

And I'm a big hot mess

Can't fit into that dress

This thing has got me I don't know

I wish it would leave but it won't let go

Second Verse

Menopause done me wrong

3 a.m. and I'm writing this song

But I'm still good to go

The next minute, low

I have sexy dreams then

Wake up and scream

Menopause done me wrong

"Meltdowns are common, as are menopausal rages," says Jane P. "Sometimes this whole thing gets too hard to handle, and our temper gets the better of us! As soon as you feel things getting out of control, protect yourself. Move to your room, take a quick drive, or go to the library so you can avoid any backlash. If there's already a situation, be quick to explain your side and listen to the other side of the disagreement so all people feel heard. Damage control is key! It will blindside you, and you will actually hear yourself saying/doing something irrational. Talk to yourself like you would your best friend and find out what you need. And then do it. Take care of yourself first."

Even Susan M., who insists menopause "hasn't been an issue at all," admits having a lack of patience. "But that's because I am simply becoming wiser and have less patience for stupidity." Susan doesn't feel it has anything to do with hormones, but rather, "it's just a matter of seeing things differently as we age."

Mother's Little Helpers

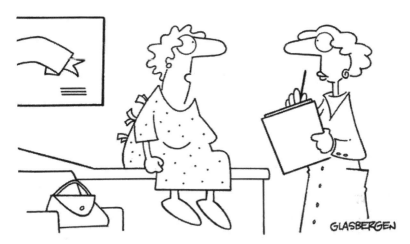

**"That pill they advertise all the time on TV.
I'm not sure what it is, but I want it!"**

Because this new (and often out of character) behavior can really start to interfere with daily life, many women turn to their doctors' prescription pads for help. Frequently, antidepressants are prescribed for anxiety, depression, and moodiness, as well as for treating hot flashes. These include Lexapro, Prozac, Paxil, and Effexor, just to name a few.

"No one touches my Prozac, or I will bite them," says Kathleen S., a self-proclaimed "Prozac princess" who says Prozac curbs at least some of her roller-coaster highs and lows.

"Why suffer?" she asks. "Why take the insanity out on the world? The people around you are usually crazy enough on a daily basis not to add to the chaos. Prozac helps soothe my emotions and gives me focus to try and grab those answers I find elusive.

"Whether it was menopause or just my crazy family, I have been on Prozac since I was 40, and over the years the level has increased to 40 milligrams a day," Kathleen says. "I believe it is the only thing helping me survive over the years."

However, for some ladies, the side effects of antidepressants make present matters worse.

Lynn B.'s doctor prescribed Pristiq (generically known as desvenlafaxine) for "taking the edge off" of her anxiety.

"I noticed a slight improvement (fewer panic attacks) after being on the meds for about four weeks," Lynn, age 57, says. "However, a new problem arose—and this had never been a problem for me before—I couldn't have an orgasm! Nothing else had changed since taking the drug, and I was puzzled. Naturally, I Googled and found I was not alone, at all. I had to make a decision: Could I live with the possibility of not having an orgasm? Or live with my anxiety? I made the decision and disposed of the pills, and I'm happy to say that my ability to orgasm has returned. I've begun meditating, and this seems to help [my anxiety]."

Dr. Angela DeRosa, author of *How Your Doctor is Slowly Killing You: A Woman's Health Survival Guide* shares her opinion on the role testosterone plays during this stage:

"Time and time again, physicians assess women's emotional changes as 'depression or anxiety.' Unfortunately, many physicians don't realize the role of testosterone in mood, and instead of getting to the root cause of their patient's anxiety, they are told to reduce their stress or placed on an anti-depressant. Testosterone is a primer of serotonin receptors in the brain. When this hormone becomes deficient, patients may experience mood changes for the first time in their lives. In patients that already have underlying mood disorders, they may become worse. Many medications contribute to testosterone deficiency, including anti-depressants, and patients need to heed caution when a doctor wants to prescribe them for symptoms that could be related to hormone deficiency or imbalance. [Antidepressants] might make patients feel better for a while, but they don't address the root cause, and ironically these medications may contribute to further testosterone deficiency. No testosterone, no orgasms, and our mood goes out the window.

Other women—some of whom rarely take anything stronger than a Motrin for a migraine—choose instead to try homeopathic remedies.

"The whole premise of natural medicine is to work *with* nature, not *against* it," says Orest Pelechaty, LAc, OMD, a doctor of Oriental Medicine who is nationally certified in acupuncture and Chinese herbal medicine and the clinic director at the *Center for Integrated Holistic Medicine* in Springfield, New Jersey. "Even if something is identical chemically, it isn't necessarily identical biochemically and especially bio-energetically.

"In some cultures, the cessation of menstruation doesn't exist as a problem, but rather, it's seen as a liberation. With no fear of pregnancy, everything is refreshed," Dr. Pelechaty notes. "'Second spring' is the Chinese way of saying menopause."

But if you haven't been following Chinese medicine for 20 years, and menopause kicks up on you, resulting in a horrific menopause instead of a "second spring," Dr. Pelechaty recommends diffusing essential oils such as jasmine, geranium, or lavender as one of the best natural remedies to help you through.

"By working through the lymphatic system, as you sniff essential oils, the brain recognizes the aromatic molecules, which act as signals that affect the entire neuro-endocrine immunological hormonal response to the organism," he explains.

Note that some oils are stinky, as they are not perfumes, but instead therapeutic agents.

Carolyn Dean, MD, ND, author of *The Magnesium Miracle,* explains the magnesium deficiency connection. "Magnesium supports our adrenal glands, which are overworked by stress, leading to combined magnesium deficiency symptoms and adrenal exhaustion symptoms of anxiety, depression, muscle weakness, fatigue, eye twitches, insomnia, anorexia, apathy, apprehension, poor memory, confusion, anger, nervousness, and rapid pulse.

"When the body is stressed—and it can be for a dozen different reasons—our magnesium reserves dump this crucial mineral into our bloodstream, and we immediately become one of those people blessed with the ability to cope. We are both calm and alert. Our friends and relatives think it's just who we are, but it's really how much magnesium we have in reserve. If the stress continues and you don't rest or replace your magnesium between episodes, your magnesium stores become depleted. Then, when you are faced with the next stressor, your stress hormones (adrenaline and cortisol) don't activate your magnesium reserves to produce a calming effect. Instead, adrenaline revs up your heart rate, elevates your blood pressure, and tenses your muscles in a fight-or-flight reaction.

"Millions of people try unsuccessfully to cope with their problems or medicate their stress with overeating, cigarettes, alcohol, street drugs, and other addictive behaviors to suppress their pain. Serotonin, the 'feel-good' brain chemical that is artificially boosted by Prozac, depends on magnesium for its production and function.

"Instead of treating stress reactions properly with magnesium, each year millions of people are introduced to the merry-go-round of psychiatric drugs and psychological counseling for symptoms that may in fact be rooted in magnesium deficiency."

Dr. Angela DeRosa notes, "Although magnesium deficiency can cause hot flashes to trigger more easily, estrogen deficiency is more likely the root cause of them. Providing estrogen balance can help reduce, or in most cases eliminate them."

Note: Whether you choose to treat hot flashes and/or depression with prescription drugs or natural remedies, it's wise to consult with your doctor first.

CHAPTER 5

Damn This Vagina!

The Last Fact of Life Mom Forgot to Mention: Vaginal Atrophy— What Is It? And Is It Treatable?

The ability to have intercourse with virtually no chance of pregnancy is one of the biggest advantages of menopause. However, just when you thought "the coast was clear," there's one little glitch. The culprit? *Atrophic vaginitis,* known more commonly as vaginal atrophy. Even more commonly known as "ouch."

During menopause, your body stops producing the hormone estrogen. As your estrogen decreases, it can cause thinning, drying, and inflammation of the vaginal walls.

Many women are so embarrassed about this symptom that they don't approach it with their doctors—or even with their closest of friends for that matter. Other women are so shocked by the change, they think it's some sort of abnormality.

Vaginal atrophy isn't a topic that comes up during casual conversation among friends. "No one ever discussed this with me," says Patricia N. age 49, "I'd never heard of it as being a part of life for so many. I thought it was an abnormality suffered by [for instance] women who'd been abused. I had no idea it could be a normal part of menopause."

The most common change in the vaginal walls is dryness. This dryness can cause friction, and friction can cause bleeding.

"Of all the things I expected would happen, never did I think I'd be as dry as the Sahara Desert down there," Pam T., age 46, says. "I cringe at the thought of even starting a relationship, not knowing if [natural lubrication] will just kick in again after a good kiss or not. I'm way too young and attractive to imagine this is how the rest of my life will be. It's so discouraging."

Slip Slidin' Away

Thankfully, over-the-counter remedies for relief from vaginal dryness can be found at your local pharmacy.

Here's the lowdown on lubricants from renowned sex and relationship educator Laura Berman, PhD, assistant clinical professor of obstetrics-gynecology and psychiatry at the Feinberg School of Medicine at Northwestern University, in Chicago:

- **Water-based lubricants:** These all-purpose lubes are the most common ones because they're safe to use with sex toys and latex contraceptives such as condoms, diaphragms, and sponges. They're easy to clean up and are formulated to be non-irritating, though some contain glycerine, which can cause yeast infections. They dry up easily, but water or saliva can quickly remedy this. Some good water-based lubricants include K-Y Ultra Gel (which has a "warming" version) and Liquid Silk. Flavored, edible water-based lubricants are also popular and fun, though they often contain yeast-encouraging sugar and glycerine.

- **Silicone-based lubricants:** These lubricants last longer than water-based ones. They can't be used with silicone sex toys because of silicone-on-silicone reactions, but you can use them with latex contraceptives and sex toys not made of silicone. Two great brands that double as sensual massage oils are Pjur Woman Bodyglide and Überlube. Keep in mind that some women are easily irritated by silicone, so test it out first. Also, silicone-based lubricants are more expensive than water-based ones. They're also harder to wash off bedding and clothing.

Another vaginal symptom is the shortening and tightening of the vaginal canal. This can be so severe it makes intercourse nearly impossible.

Helene R., age 57, describes her vagina as being "like an abandoned house with a locked, stuck door and cobwebs everywhere—dried up and blown away. I haven't let anything in there for years."

Diane Z., age 59, had always enjoyed what she considered a healthy sex life before menopause; however, sex was almost exclusively oral. But with the prospect of zero chance of an unwanted pregnancy, she was happy to finally engage in all the intercourse her husband wanted after Aunt Flo's permanent departure when she was around age 49.

"I was ready and willing, but apparently, not able!" Diane says. "It was like I was sealed shut! An awful thought ran through my mind: *Was it possible that my vagina had actually closed up from the lack of intercourse?* I immediately went to my doctor, who assured me this was not the case. As I lay on the examining table, he said, 'Well, I got in!' "Yes, I said, but you're using tools!"

Could lack of intercourse have been the culprit? Is there some kind of "use it or lose it" rule?

Doctors sometimes prescribe hormone replacement therapy (HRT) or estrogen replacement therapy (ERT). The hormones are distributed through gels, sprays, and patches; taken orally; or dispensed via intravaginal creams.

"Estrogen deficiency causes the vaginal tissues to become thin and fragile versus thick and plump," Dr. DeRosa notes. "This leads to vaginal dryness, itching and burning as well as painful intercourse. Hormone replacement therapy treats the root cause of this and can be used safely in the majority of women."

"In menopause, a woman lacks estrogen because there are no longer any more eggs in the ovaries," explains Marlan Schwartz, MD, past chairman of the department of obstetrics and gynecology at Robert Wood Johnson University Hospital, in Somerset, New Jersey. "Replacing estrogen is the goal. If the woman has a uterus, because unopposed estrogen on the uterus can cause a problem (primarily potentially cancer) if used for a period of time (usually at least five years), we add progesterone to counter the effects of the estrogen on the uterus. If the woman does not have a uterus, only estrogen is needed.

"The large Women's Health Initiative (WHI) compared estrogen (E) to estrogen and progesterone (EP), specifically the estrogen in Premarin and the progesterone in Prempro (medroxyprogesterone)," Dr. Schwartz continues. "The progesterone is different from ones used in birth control pills. Basically, for breast cancer, they found in every 10,000 women, those with EP had eight more breast cancers than expected (which is not statistically significant) and seven fewer breast cancers in the E group. The average age in that study was 64. If you extrapolate out to women ages 50 to 59, you find there's much benefit to estrogen [use]."

There are many benefits for women going on HRT especially if it is within 10 years of menopause," says Dr. DeRosa. "But the benefits after 10 years become more neutral."

However, some women are adamantly opposed to estrogen replacement therapy due to its potential health risks or side effects.

"No thank you!" says comedienne *Robin Fox*. "I'm taking a shot of vodka and choose to have a lot more sex with Wolfie. I'm hoping to make calluses like I did when learning to play the guitar."

Many lesbian couples cope with the problem simply by ceasing the use of dildos.

While today's liberated women "of a certain age" may feel comfortable talking about vaginal atrophy with close friends (usually after a glass or two of wine), the condition is not typically a subject that comes up with much younger women—unless you share a history of hysterectomies.

Patricia N., age 48, confided in a neighbor. The conversation went like this: "I want to tell you something, and I don't want you to look at me funny. I think my vagina is broken.

"I told her how I feel normal and happy and I like men (not currently dating), but it just doesn't act the same anymore," Patricia says. "My neighbor admitted the same to me. We're attractive, generally healthy, I get hit on all the time, and I enjoy some eye candy, but never in my wildest dreams did I think at this age I'd be here."

Kathleen S. had a partial hysterectomy at age 26. "Things went okay for quite a while, but then as the symptoms began, my doctor put me on estrogen and eventually [estrogen] with testosterone called Estratest, a single pill once a day. This worked great for years; it kept the symptoms away and allowed me a fairly normal sex life. However, articles came out that HRT was dangerous for certain types of cancer and/or heart problems, and all my girlfriends, plus a new doctor, advised stopping the medicine. Big mistake. Menopause roared through and sex became extremely painful. It took about six to nine months to get it through my husband's head that it hurt to the point of 'Don't touch me!' Plus, I actually bled a few times as the skin inside tore.

"I tried a vaginal cream, but it was more bother than effective," Kathleen continues. "I leaked in the morning, and it helped the pain some, a little but not enough to try sex again. I am one of those women who after 55 can just live without sex, I'm done. It was fun while it lasted, but it became another chore like washing dishes. And then with the pain, I just quit. But my husband has whined for years, 'I'm too young to give up sex.' So I went to several doctors, all women, and most of them said it was my choice and they didn't recommend starting anything at my age. I was too old to go back on HRT.

"Then I had a younger female doctor who suggested a patch called Vivelle-Dot with estrogen," Kathleen says. "I definitely knew something was going on because my mood swings were back in full force and my breasts were tender. I'm a fairly quiet person, so when I found myself snapping at people at work and yelling at my grandsons, I went back to the doctor and she added progesterone pills at night to balance the mood swings. This was not a fix-all, and after numerous unsuccessful attempts at sex, I stopped the medication once and for all."

Some women do report improvement with the use of vaginal creams such as Estrace. Others, like Cindy W., age 58, give up intercourse altogether and enjoy a perfectly mutually happy exclusively oral sex life. "It's a win-win for me and my hubby," Cindy says. "He's happy he can still make me happy, and truth be know, I've always preferred oral sex anyway."

Making love used to make my toes curl. Now it gives me foot cramps.

—Kathy Dice, Comedienne

CHAPTER 6

Speaking of Sex

Libido: Lost and Found

Like many perimenopausal or menopausal women, Christine D., age 50, concedes that for many months, she lost almost all interest in sex. "For close to an entire year, I was just as content to snuggle in bed with my husband, and nothing more. Then, one day, I don't know what happened, but I guess I got my mojo back."

"I don't know what the proper name is to describe my feeling toward lovemaking right now, but I think it's 'asexual,'" says Mary D., age 53.

"It's a rough situation, not wanting sex in my relationship," Sandra, age 62, notes. "I think if we were in a better situation financially in our pre-retirement years, it would be grounds for divorce. For years, I have pushed away from snuggling in the bedroom because of fear it would lead to sex, and I'd have to say no. Over the years, it has made my husband more grouchy, irritable, and difficult to live with."

"Once my husband realized that my stripping off my nightgown at night didn't mean he was about to 'get lucky,' he started to roll over and start snoring," says Carol G. "Things changed a few months later when I began to feel as sexually excited as a much younger woman, which has continued through the years."

A *Reader's Digest* article on *the Truth About Sex After 50* differentiates fact from fiction. Here are two of my favorites.

Fiction: Beyond a certain age, people have little interest in sex.

Fact: There is no age limit on sexuality, but for people age 50 and over, sexual satisfaction depends more on the overall quality of the relationship than it does for younger couples. A National Council on Aging survey reports that among people age 60 and over who have regular intercourse, 74 percent of the men and 70 percent of the women find their sex lives more satisfying than when they were in their forties.

Fiction: A woman loses her ability to have orgasms as she ages.

Fact: Many women find increased sexual pleasure after menopause, including more frequent or more intense orgasms.

Essential Oils:
You Make Me Feel Like a Natural Woman

Menopausal women might find help in a bottle—an essential oil bottle, that is. One essential oil that has desire-boosting benefits is jasmine.

Orest Pelechaty, LAc, OMD, a doctor of Oriental Medicine suggests that after several weeks of diffusing jasmine essential oil, "you might find yourself getting friskier."

"The problem with naturopathic medicine is that it usually takes a long time to get profound changes—because the healing is very gradual, which requires diligence," Dr. Pelechaty says. "The upside is that it's very safe and gentle. It's not like we're going to stimulate some gland; it's a very different approach than Western medicine."

Dr. Pelechaty notes that holistic medicine looks at the bigger picture. "We strive for a harmonious balance and look at natural ways to rebuild, regenerate, and harmonize."

Chinese medicine is based on common sense and direct sensory perception. "We don't add all these layers of complexity between a phenomenon and a person. It's all very commonsense stuff. It's very direct and doesn't require a lot of theorizing," he says.

Dr. Pelechaty also recommends diffusing the essential oil ylang ylang (pronounced eee-lang eee-lang), which has been known to induce a relaxed feeling.

"Chinese medicine has its own language," Dr. Pelechaty says. "It's much more 'software' rather than 'hardware.' It has a lot of poetic language because it speaks more to the human experience. If someone is anxious and can't sleep, in Chinese medicine, we refer to this as 'the heart spirit is not in the palace.' Here we are really talking more about the spiritual heart, how to calm the spirit. When you have a more calm heart and your dreams are happier, you might have better connection with your body, with your relationships, and with your environment, which may lead to a healthier sexual response."

It's important to note that there is a lack of industry standards and regulations on terminology such as *natural* or *pure*. Even though an essential oil is labeled "GRAS" (Generally Regarded As Safe), that doesn't guarantee purity. Many essential oils sold in health food stores or pharmacies may contain ingredients that are unsafe for topical use. Dr. Pelechaty recommends essential oils from *www.youngliving.com*.

Use essential oils with extreme caution, and always consult with a knowledgeable health practitioner or your physician if there is any uncertainty about proper usage.

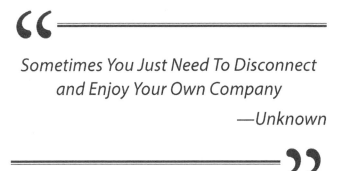

*Sometimes You Just Need To Disconnect
and Enjoy Your Own Company*

—*Unknown*

She Bop

Some women who have lost the desire for sex with their partners still want to orgasm on their own.

The *Reader's Digest* article mentioned earlier in this chapter noted, "Masturbation can increase sexual pleasure, both with and without a partner, for women. It helps keep vaginal tissues moist and elastic and boosts hormone levels, which fuels sex drive."

Judy M., age 61, shared, "Once in a while it's a nice way to relax before going to sleep and while my husband is out in the living room still watching television. I can make the magic happen in minutes. I know where my spot is and what it needs."

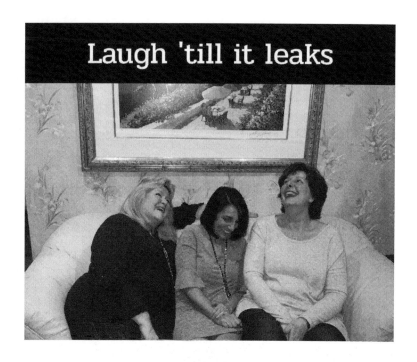

Oops, Urine Trouble Again!

Because of the thinning of the vaginal walls, menopausal women may also be prone to bothersome urinary incontinence.

Sometime around the age of 49, Connie T. couldn't even take a walk around the block without wearing a panty liner made for urine leakage.

"It became very annoying," Connie says. "No amount of Kegel exercises helped." Eventually, she opted for a surgical procedure known as a bladder sling.

"Essentially, it is a hernia involving the neck of the bladder (at origin of urethra), and whenever you cough, laugh, sneeze, etc., there is a little movement at the neck—anything that increases intra-abdominal pressure and puts a strain (or stress) on the neck of the bladder."

"There are different forms of urinary incontinence," explains Marlan Schwartz, MD, past chairman of the department of obstetrics and gynecology at Robert Wood Johnson University Hospital, in Somerset, New Jersey. "Stress incontinence happens when a few drops of urine leak out when laughing, coughing, or sneezing. Urge incontinence, also known as overactive bladder, comes with the strong, sudden, uncontrollable urge to urinate."

Stress urinary incontinence is a common problem. It affects 15 to 35 percent of the population over the age of 60. And it affects women twice as often as men.

To diagnose the type of urinary incontinence, a doctor might recommend a urinalysis, a bladder stress test, or an ultrasound.

The first-line treatment for urinary incontinence is usually Kegel exercises.

"Kegels are commonly tried because they're cheap (free), and one can do them any time," Their effectiveness is relatively low because they must be done multiple times daily and continued indefinitely. It's like lifting weights to get muscles; once you stop ....

"Other treatments include biofeedback, bladder training, and dietary changes/restrictions. Some medicines help reduce the number of leaking episodes one has. But, of course, wetting yourself only five times a day instead of eight times still leaves you wet."

The definitive treatment for urinary incontinence is a bladder neck suspension procedure, which is typically a same-day procedure that takes less than a half hour with usually a pretty quick recovery."

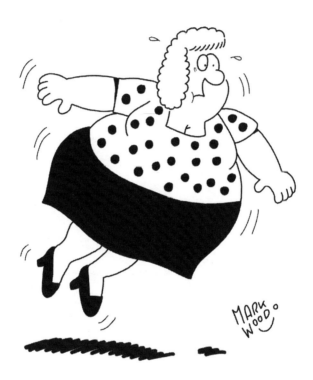

Maureen had experienced sudden bouts of bloat before, but nothing like this.

7

Foods That Trigger and Foods That Suppress Menopause Symptoms

Weighing in on What to Eat, What to Avoid

During periods of fluctuating hormones, especially throughout menstruation, many women report they crave chocolate. Considering the amount of hormones fluctuating during menopause and the added stress other symptoms cause, is it any wonder that menopausal women crave chocolate too?

One possible explanation is offered by Emerita, a woman's health blog.

"[During menstruation], as ovulation occurs and estrogen fluctuates, so do your other hormones. The body reacts by trying to balance out the hormones.

Cortisol, the stress hormone, often increases. Serotonin, on the other hand, known as the feel-good hormone, can be increased by exercise, as well as by eating some foods. You may crave simple carbs, sugars, and fats when serotonin is low, as these foods can elevate serotonin quickly—and briefly. Chocolate is a similar but unique beast. It is thought women specifically crave chocolate due to its ability to mimic serotonin and release endorphins, which may decrease depression and anxiety. Some theories cite the chemical phenylethylamine, or PEA, which is found in chocolate and stimulates blood pressure and increases heart rate."

Sage Advice

One staple in the kitchen that is a must-have for women in menopause is sage. It's particularly useful for digestion.

"As we age, our digestion degenerates," says Orest Pelechaty, LAc, OMD, a doctor of Oriental Medicine who is nationally certified in acupuncture and Chinese herbal medicine and the clinic director at the *Center for Integrated Holistic Medicine* in Springfield, New Jersey."[In Chinese medicine], we rebuild it by using bitters. Sage is one such bitter, and it's a phenomenal medicine with a variety of side uses. Besides adding it to turkey, sage has a lot of applications, one of which is to break the pattern of excessive sweating. It's also good for mental fatigue, hair loss, or depression. And you can grow it in a pot in your kitchen."

Some women claim sage tea quells hot flashes. Sage tea is easy to make, and it's worth a try. *Julie Dargan*, a registered nurse, naturopath BHSc, speaker, author, and menopause consultant at www.menopausewhisperer.com, says, "The use of sage as a natural remedy for excessive sweating and hot flashes has its roots in traditional folk medicine. Sage tea has a longstanding reputation for lifting the spirits as well as being touted as an excellent remedy for impaired memory."

To make, Dargan says, "Simply steep 5 to 10 fresh sage leaves in teapot of boiling water fresh off the boil. Steep for 5 to 10 minutes before serving. No milk or sugar need to be added."

The Weight-Menopause Connection

*I swear I'm not eating again—ever.
After tomorrow night's dinner with
friends. No, wait, after Saturday's lunch
with family. Oh, I forgot—Saturday
night dinner with friends. After that,
I swear. Oh … never mind … fat and
happy. Pass the chips and dip!*

—Debbie H.

If you're overweight, you can minimize menopausal symptoms and reduce the long-term risks of declining hormones by losing weight, says Mary Jane Minkin, MD, clinical professor of obstetrics, gynecology, and reproductive sciences at Yale University School of Medicine, in New Haven, Connecticut.

Slimming down reduces the risks of heart disease and breast cancer, both of which go up after menopause, says Dr. Minkin. *New research* shows that it may also help overweight or obese women cut down on hot flashes.

"About 100 percent of my patients going through menopause complain of bloating," Dr. Minkin says.

"Although the reasons aren't clear, fluctuating hormones during perimenopause may play a role."

Dr. Minkin recommends cutting the amount of salt and processed carbohydrates in your diet because they can make you retain water. But don't skimp on whole grains, which are rich in heart-healthy fiber, or on fruits and vegetables.

I've gained five pounds and nothing is going down weight wise. I've graduated to a size 6 from a size 2, even though I work out and watch my diet. I have a spare tire!

—Roxanne R.

Foods high in high-fructose corn syrup and white breads have been known to be big contributors to belly fat. Even some granola is so loaded with sugar, you might be better off eating that chocolate bar, so read packages carefully and note the sugar content.

In my younger days, I had a flat tummy and a large rear end. Now, I have a flat rear end and big tummy. It's as if my buttocks moved from my behind to my front.

—Beverly N.

Most juices made from concentrate have just as much sugar as soda does, or sometimes even more, because fiber is eliminated in the fruit juice concentration process.

Also bad for belly fat are trans fats, such as those found in margarine.

Orest Pelechaty, LAc, OMD, notes the importance of fat in your diet.

"If you are deficient in cholesterol, you cannot build hormones," Dr. Pelechaty says. "Fat actually can be good for you, provided it comes from seed oil—not commercial burgers."

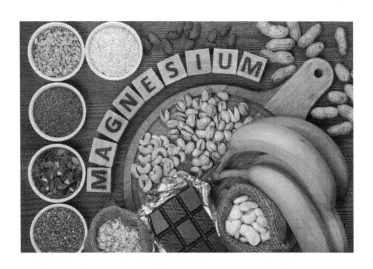

Magnesium to the Rescue, Again!

One mineral that's common in many foods that can ease menopausal symptoms is magnesium.

"Unfortunately, unless the soil that vegetables are being grown in is re-mineralized, most soil is depleted of magnesium," says Carolyn Dean, MD, ND, a medical advisory board member of the Nutritional Magnesium Association at www.nutritionalmagne-sium.org. "People following a raw food, green drink, organic diet get just as magnesium-deficient with leg cramps and heart palpitations as a result."

One way to get more magnesium, Dr. Dean says, is to start your day with this simple-to-prepare beverage: Upon rising, combine the juice of half to one whole fresh lemon with warm water. Sweeten with stevia if desired. Enjoy the beverage warm.

Or for breakfast, try her Crockpot Cereal.

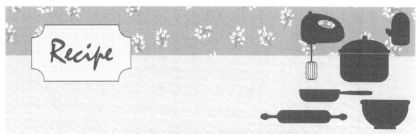

Crockpot Cereal

What You'll Need:

Choose two grains from the following: buckwheat, millet, rye, oats, amaranth, or quinoa

Choose one seed from the following: sunflower seeds or pumpkin seeds

Choose one nut from the following: almonds, cashews, filberts, walnuts, or pecans

Fresh or frozen blueberries, strawberries, raspberries, banana, peach, or pear

Flaxseed oil, organic butter, or fresh ground flaxseeds.

Rice milk, almond milk, or soy milk (optional)

Wheat germ (optional)

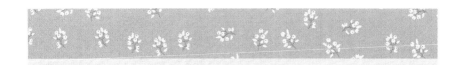

How to Make It:

For each serving, combine 2 ounces of dry mixture, including nuts and seeds, with 5 ounces of water in a 1-quart slow cooker.

Cook overnight on low for 6 to 8 hours. In the morning, place in a bowl, add 2 to 4 ounces of fruit per serving, and stir to combine. Add 2 tablespoons of flaxseed oil, 1 tablespoon of organic butter, or 2 tablespoons of ground flaxseeds (ground fresh in a coffee grinder).

You may add rice milk, almond milk, or small amounts of soy milk as needed. For extra magnesium, sprinkle on wheat germ (kept in the freezer).

Substitutions:

1. Instead of using a slow cooker, you can soak 2 ounces of grain mixture overnight in 5 ounces of water, with or without 2 tablespoons of plain yogurt or kefir (refrigerate if using the yogurt or kefir). In the morning, bring the mixture to a boil, reduce the heat, and simmer on low for 20 minutes. You may have to add more water to avoid dryness. Serve with 2 tablespoons ground flaxseeds (ground fresh in a coffee grinder).

2. Instead of soaking overnight, combine 2 ounces of grain mixture with 6 ounces of water. Bring to a boil, reduce the heat, and simmer for 30 minutes.

Dr. Dean recommends the following for lunch or dinnertime meals.

- Brown rice and vegetables, cooked with 2 ounces of dulse or other sea vegetables

- Leafy green salad, soup with added sea vegetables, and Essene sprouted bread or Ezekiel bread

- Fish, greens (collards, spinach, Swiss chard), and salad

- Egg omelet with sautéed vegetables

- Chicken with vegetables

- Soup with sea vegetables and salad

- Stir-fried grains (use leftover grains from breakfast, if you have them) and vegetables

- Roasted vegetables with wild rice

- Salad with cooked organic legumes (kidney beans, lentils, black beans, pinto beans, chickpeas)

- Wheat-free pasta (rice, spelt, kamut) with pesto, tomato sauce, and green vegetables

- Mixed salad with avocado

Also be sure to choose snacks rich in magnesium, including raw vegetables, dried fruit (prunes and figs), shelled nuts and seeds (raw, not processed or salted), baked blue corn chips, or popcorn.

Sip on drinks such as pure clean water, green tea, freshly squeezed lemon juice and water, or cranberry juice sweetened with stevia.

Keep It Simple

"There's no one size fits all when it comes to diet," says Elizabeth Girouard, a certified integrated nutrition health coach at www.puresimplewellness.com.

To keep healthy and reduce stress, cravings, and midday energy slumps, Girouard recommends eating pure, simple whole foods found in nature with a focus on an anti-inflammatory regime.

"Herbs can help the body with reducing inflammation," Girouard says. "Try incorporating 1/2 teaspoon of herbs, such as cloves, ginger, rosemary, turmeric, oregano, and cinnamon, into your daily menus."

Herbs are a great way to add flavor and health benefits to your food with no additional calories.

"Drinking plenty of water is also key," Girouard adds. "A good rule of thumb is to drink half of your body weight in ounces. But don't start all at once. Build up to it. Studies have shown that when your body is well hydrated, it can boost your metabolism up to 30 percent. When you are slightly dehydrated, as little as 1 to 2 percent, it can increase your stress hormones. This causes us to store more belly fat and also to crave more sugar."

Girouard, who has made a business out of preparing and delivering gourmet healthy meals from *www.zingmeals.com,* also recommends, "Strive for 10 servings of fruit and vegetables per day, with [a ratio of] three vegetables to one fruit. Avocados, in particular, are a great source of healthy fat, fiber, and protein.

"Fiber is very important to 'keep the system going.' If you are not having at least one bowel movement per day, you are probably not eating enough fiber and drinking enough water," she says. "A healthier lifestyle doesn't have to mean dramatic, overnight change. Make small, consistent changes for long-term results. For example, start by replacing your sugary breakfast cereal with steel-cut oats or a vegetable and fruit smoothie."

Here are a few simple, delicious smoothie recipes:

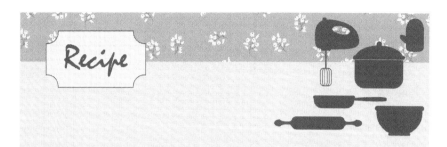

Choco-Cherry Smoothie

What You'll Need:

- 1 to 2 cups spinach or other leafy greens
- 1 cup frozen cherries
- 1 to 2 cups filtered water (depending on desired consistency)
- 2 tablespoons chia seeds
- 1 heaping tablespoon raw cacao powder
- Pinch of cinnamon
- A few drops of stevia or other healthy sweetener (optional)

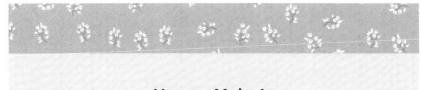

How to Make It:

In a high-speed blender, add all of the ingredients, putting the softer items on the bottom.

Start the blender on low and slowly move up to high, using the tamper as needed to include ingredients into the blending process. Blend for 45 to 60 seconds, or until smooth.

This recipe is great for breakfast, an afternoon snack, or a sweet treat. You can substitute berries or bananas for the cherries.

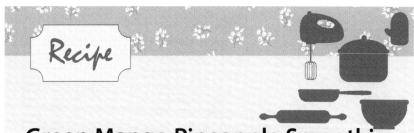

Green Mango Pineapple Smoothie

What You'll Need:

- 1 to 2 cups spinach or other leafy greens
- 1 cup frozen pineapple
- 1 cup frozen mango
- 1 cup filtered water
- Ice (optional, if not using frozen fruit)
- Raw honey or stevia (optional)

How to Make It:

In a high-speed blender, add all of the ingredients, putting the softer items on the bottom.

Start the blender on low and slowly move up to high, using the tamper as needed to include ingredients into the blending process. If using ice, add water as needed to reach the desired consistency. Blend for 45 to 60 seconds, or until smooth.

Another option is to replace your sugary afternoon snack with hummus and carrots, which contains protein, healthy fat, and fiber for a more sustained release of energy. Avoiding refined sugar and all processed foods is key to keeping your weight down. All calories are not created equal. Read the package. If you can't pronounce the ingredients in a food, don't eat it, unless, of course, it's quinoa.

Say Yes to Soy

Soy contains plant estrogens, so many women think it can increase their breast cancer risk, says Dr. Minkin. However, there is little data to support this. The misconception likely comes from studies of high-dose soy supplements, which may stimulate the growth of estrogen-sensitive tumors.

Soy foods such as tofu, soy nuts, and soy milk may offer relief from mild hot flashes and are not thought to increase breast cancer risk.

"Women in Japan have the highest soy intake and the lowest risk of breast cancer, but Japanese women who move to the United States and eat less soy have a higher risk," adds Dr. Minkin.

Cheers? To Menopause!

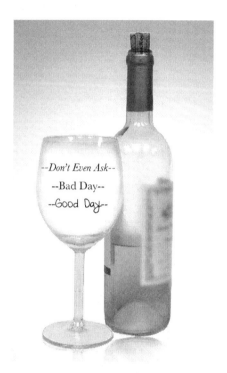

While many women of a certain age turn to wine to take the edge off a particularly stressful day, alcohol and menopause don't always mix. In fact, alcohol may actually trigger hot flashes.

"I had one sip of champagne at a wedding to toast the bride and groom and went into a full-body sweat," says Haralee W., 62, "I had to leave the wedding because I was in a vintage silk dress that was sticking to me!"

Many menopausal women also complain of migraines almost immediately after drinking.

That doesn't mean you can't enjoy a few drinks once in a while. But "moderation" can mean different things to different people. According to *The North American Menopause Society, Drink to Your Health at Menopause, or Not?*, this is how the National Institute on Alcohol Abuse and Alcoholism (NIAAA) defines the amounts of consumption, and the respective good and bad points of drinking alcohol in menopause:

The National Institute on Alcohol Abuse and Alcoholism (NIAAA) defines one standard drink as:

- 5 fluid ounces of wine (about 12 percent alcohol) (Don't let your wine glass fool you. Most hold much more than 5 ounces.)
- 12 fluid ounces (usually one can or bottle) of regular beer (about 5 percent alcohol)
- 1.5 fluid ounces (one shot) of 80-proof distilled spirits

This is how the NIAAA defines different levels of drinking for women:

- Moderate (low risk): no more than seven drinks per week and no more than three drinks on any single day

- Heavy (at-risk): consuming more than the moderate daily or weekly amounts
- Binge drinking: drinking so much within about two hours that your blood alcohol level reaches 0.08 g/dL (about four drinks)

How much is good?

- Moderate drinkers have a significantly lower risk of coronary heart disease than nondrinkers. The heart benefits of moderate drinking become apparent at menopause when heart disease risk normally goes up, and the heart benefits continue after that. Hormone therapy doesn't affect that benefit.
- Women who drink moderately have a lower risk of type 2 diabetes.
- Those who drink moderate amounts of alcohol, especially wine, have a lower risk of dementia than those who don't drink at all.
- Women who drink lightly or moderately have a lower risk of stroke than nondrinkers.
- At and after menopause (ages 50 to 62), women who drink moderately have stronger bones than nondrinkers.

- Midlife and older women who drink moderately have a lower risk of becoming obese than nondrinkers.

How much is bad?

- Any amount of alcohol increases the risk of breast cancer. The increase in risk is there, but small, for women who drink one drink a day. Women who drink two to five drinks a day have about 1.5 times the risk of nondrinkers. (The increased risk doesn't seem to have anything to do with alcohol's effect on estrogen levels.)
- Drinking alcohol increases the risk of many other cancers. The risk rises with the amount of alcohol consumed. (And the risk rises higher if you smoke as well.)
- Drinking may trigger hot flashes for some women, although that isn't based in research. So determine whether it's a personal trigger for you. (As for a general risk of experiencing hot flashes and night sweats, some studies find alcohol increases it, whereas others find the opposite.)
- Alcohol has harmful interactions with many medications, even ones you may not think about, such as medicines for arthritis, indigestion or heartburn, high cholesterol, and high blood pressure. Check out which ones

here: https://pubs.niaaa.nih.gov/publications/ Medicine/medicine.htm.

- More than moderate drinking increases the risk of cardiovascular disease. Among heavy drinkers, women are more susceptible to alcohol-related heart disease than men.

- Women who drink heavily are prone to central obesity—the apple shape that is a big risk for cardiovascular disease.

- Heavy drinking can lead to osteoporosis that cannot be reversed. It's also a risk for fractures.

- Binge drinking increases the risk of developing type 2 diabetes.

- Women at menopause are especially vulnerable to depression, and heavy drinking can just make that worse. Heavy drinking itself can lead to depression, and women who show signs of alcoholism are two to seven times more at risk of developing depression than men.

- Alcoholic women are more susceptible than men to key organ system damage, including heart muscle damage, nerve damage, cirrhosis, and possibly brain damage as well.

The take-home message? If you drink alcohol, enjoy yourself, but make sure your drinking is moderate.

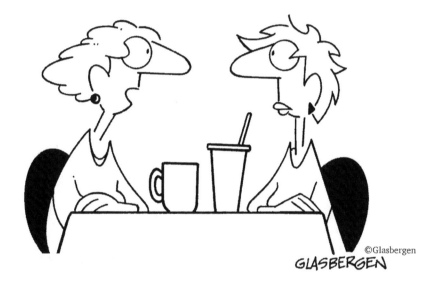

"My bones are getting softer, but my arteries
are getting harder, so it balances out!"

CHAPTER 8

Bone Loss: It's Not Humerus!

Facts and Fractures

Being female puts us at risk of developing osteoporosis and broken bones. Here are some facts on *What Women Need to Know* (reprinted with permission from the *National Osteoporosis Foundation*, Arlington Va 22022. All rights reserved.)

- Of the estimated 10 million Americans with osteoporosis, about eight million, or 80 percent, are women.

- Approximately one in two women over age 50 will break a bone because of osteoporosis.

- A woman's risk of breaking a hip is equal to her combined risk of breast, uterine, and ovarian cancer.

Estrogen, a hormone in women that protects bones, decreases sharply when we reach menopause, which can cause bone loss. This is why the chance of developing osteoporosis increases as women reach menopause. For some women, this bone loss is rapid and severe. Two major factors that affect your chance of getting osteoporosis are:

The amount of bone you have when you reach menopause. The greater your bone density is to begin with, the lower your chance of developing osteoporosis. If you had low peak bone mass or other risk factors that caused you to lose bone, your chance of getting osteoporosis is greater.

How fast you lose bone after you reach menopause. For some women, bone loss happens faster than for others. In fact, a woman can lose up to 20 percent of her bone density during the five to seven years following menopause. If you lose bone quickly, you have a greater chance of developing osteoporosis.

What about taking estrogen?

If you have menopausal symptoms, such as hot flashes, your healthcare provider may prescribe estrogen therapy (ET) or estrogen with progesterone hormone therapy (HT). In addition to controlling your menopausal symptoms, these therapies can also help prevent bone loss. Some women are advised not to take ET or HT because of the possible increased risks for breast cancer, strokes, heart attacks, blood clots, and cognitive (mental) decline. It's important to discuss the risks and benefits of your treatment options with your healthcare provider.

Bone density testing:

A bone density test shows the amount of bone a person has in the hip, spine, or other bones. It is routinely recommended for postmenopausal women and men age 50 and older and is how osteoporosis is diagnosed in older people. Bone density tests are usually done for premenopausal women only if they break several bones easily or break bones that are unusual for their age, such as bones in the hip or spine. Also, if you have a condition or take a medicine that causes secondary osteoporosis, your healthcare provider may order a bone density test. This test should be done on a DXA machine. DXA (or DEXA) stands for dual energy X-ray absorptiometry.

One or two years after an initial bone density test, your doctor may choose to do a second bone density test to determine if you have low peak bone mass that is staying the same or if you are losing bone. If your bone density drops significantly between the first and second test, you may be losing bone and further evaluation by a healthcare provider is needed.

Understanding your bone density test results:

A bone density test result shows a Z-score and a T-score. T-scores are used to diagnose osteoporosis in postmenopausal women and men age 50 and older, but not in premenopausal women. A Z-score compares your bone density to what is normal for someone your age. While a Z-score alone is not used to diagnose osteoporosis in premenopausal women, it can provide important information.

If your Z-score is above -2.0, your bone density is considered within the ranges expected for your age, or normal, according to the International Society for Clinical Densitometry (ISCD). For example, a Z-score of +0.5, -0.5, and -1.5 is considered normal for most premenopausal women.

If your Z-score is -2.0 or lower, your bone density is considered below the expected range. Examples are -2.1, -2.3, and -2.5. If your Z-score is in this range, your healthcare provider will consider your health history and possible causes of bone loss, including secondary osteoporosis, before making a diagnosis of osteoporosis.

If your Z-score is normal, but you've broken one or more bones from a minor injury, your healthcare provider may diagnose you with osteoporosis because some people with normal bone density break bones easily. As mentioned above, a bone density test will also show a T-score. A T-score compares bone density to what is normal in a healthy 30-year-old adult.

"A prescription drug may be prescribed when there is enough bone loss to present a significant chance of a fracture," says Marlan Schwartz, MD, past chairman of the department of obstetrics and gynecology at Robert Wood Johnson University Hospital, in Somerset, New Jersey. "This would be based upon the results of a bone density screening, as well as other risk factors, such as medical conditions or medicines that you are taking."

Don't Get Bone Loss in the First Place!

Regular exercise and a diet rich in calcium can help thwart the onset of bone loss. "Recently, much discussion has centered on how effective calcium and vitamin D are in preventing osteoporosis," notes Dr. Schwartz. "Generally speaking, one should get about 1,200 milligrams (in divided doses) of calcium per day, ideally from food sources. (We can absorb about 500 milligrams at one time.) Then supplements come in. As to vitamin D, it seems everyone in the world is low in vitamin D. The best to take is D3, and the latest advice is to take 2,000 IU per day. Vitamin D is fat soluble and can be stored in your fat cells, so you can take a larger amount at one time and take it less often, for example, 14,000 IU (which may be seven pills) once per week.

"Weight-bearing exercise, which can be as simple as walking, is a good thing to do to help prevent osteoporosis. Having said that, it is not effective for everyone, and if you have been doing that and *still* have bone loss, that isn't doing it for you—much like the runner who is in great shape and has a heart attack—I'd still have the angioplasty," cautions Dr. Schwartz.

Unfortunately, despite these dietary measures and engaging in weight-bearing exercise, heredity does still put many women at risk.

Osteopenia, Osteoporosis Meds: When Diet and Exercise Aren't Enough

There are various classes of medicines available for the prevention or treatment of osteopenia or osteoporosis, notes Dr. Schwartz. Bisphosphonates, selective estrogen receptor modifiers (SERMs), and estrogen are used for both osteopenia and osteoporosis. Other medications, such as RANK ligand inhibitors are used for osteoporosis only. Bisphosphonates include Fosamax (taken daily or weekly), Boniva (taken monthly), Actonel (taken weekly or monthly), and Atelvia (taken weekly); most of these have generics as well.

SERMs include Evista, which is a daily pill that is also indicated to prevent breast cancer. Estrogens, either oral or transdermal, also help prevent osteoporosis.

Those for only osteoporosis include a bisphosphonate injectable called Reclast (taken every 1 to 2 years) and RANK ligand inhibitors, such as Prolia, a subcutaneous injection given twice a year.

Joann R., age 57, elected to go with a daily bone medicine. "It's easier to remember to take it once a day, and if I have to take an important supplement every day, it also reminds me to take my multivitamins and calcium such as *TheraCal™ D2000*. Weekly pill containers are not just for old people!"

Dr. Schwartz cautions, "All medicines have side effects and contraindications, and these are often specific to the drug or class of drug. So, for oral bisphosphonates, risks include GI reflux or ulcer disease, [and these] would be reasons to not take these. Also, kidney disease is a problem for most of these meds. For estrogen, there are other risks to that class of drugs. For Evista, increased risk of DVT [deep vein thrombosis] would be a reason to not take it; if you have a breast cancer history, you should check with your doctor."

"*Out of clutter, find simplicity.*"

—*Albert Einstein*

CHAPTER 9

Nesting, Part Deux

Prior to giving birth, many women experience a phenomenon called nesting. The desire to have everything just right before the new arrival is prefaced by a sudden newfound burst of energy to clean and organize. So is it any wonder that during a time of intense hormonal fluctuations, menopausal women take housekeeping to an entirely new level too?

By the time we're in our late forties or early fifties, chances are, we all end up with a lot of stuff. Even if we are "neatniks," the time may come when our parents and other family or friends pass away and we're forced into accumulating even more possessions.

If you've ever had to dismantle a home for a deceased loved one, it may have become evident that you don't want your own family to go through the same chore of finding a place for all of your belongings. If you have grown children who have finally left the nest, chances are they left behind whatever wouldn't fit into their new place, and you (willing or not) became the designated caretaker of all the things they couldn't seem to part with. One day, many women get:

The Urge to Purge

Downsizing into smaller living quarters, where space is limited, can provide a real jump start.

"When it came time to downsize and move to our retirement home, I realized, sadly, none of the kids will want china, crystal, silverware, and 150 table-Cloths! Jane P., 62, says. "There is little sentimentality over keepsakes, and so I ruthlessly donated or tossed many articles that will never be missed by anyone other than me. It felt somewhat liberating to have less 'stuff' to care for and store."

How can you get rid of the stuff? Facebook, Craigslist, Freecycle, EBay, and Etsy provide many ways in which to sell or give away.

An only child, Patricia N., age 49, grew up in New York. "My father died when I was six years old, and I lived with my mother in New York City until her death when I was in my twenties. I suffered from endometriosis, which led to a partial hysterectomy.

"New York is very expensive, and I eventually moved to a cute apartment in New Jersey, which was also expensive," Patricia says. "I always just felt like that was my lot in life. Where else was I going to go? I figured one day I'd get married and move with my husband. It wasn't until 2013 that I decided to 'stop the madness.'

"I own my own business and work from home, so I could do what I do anywhere in the world. I realized the only thing that had kept me tied to my apartment was my stuff. The $5,000 wall unit, the crystal wine decanters I'd collected all those years, things that would cost a fortune to pick up and move somewhere else. I donated everything I owned, including suits I'd never wear again (sizes 2 through 4; I'm a size 8 now) and even pots and pans to the Lupus Foundation, and the rest I put on Freecycle. I packed up and moved to North Carolina, knowing not a soul. It's the most freeing, cleansing thing I've ever done."

Japanese cleaning consultant Marie Kondo takes tidying up to a whole new level in her bestselling book, *The Life-Changing Magic of Tidying Up: The Japanese Art of Decluttering and Organizing.* Her "Kon-Mari" method provides detailed guidance for determining what items spark joy (and which don't), and the subsequent decluttering has helped her followers enjoy the magic of an orderly home. But for some menopausal women, joy seems to be attached to less and less, and they purge with reckless abandon.

Lauren B., the self-proclaimed "Boss of Toss," went on a purging binge that lasted about six years. "I woke up one day and decided that I no longer had any attachment to most 'things' in my home. I literally went into each room on a daily basis and collected items that were no longer associated with any feelings. Only the most precious of my children's art projects were saved. I tried to be extremely rational (which should have been my first clue that something was wrong). But let's face it, glittered and glued dry macaroni collages last only so long.

"At one point, I thought I'd lost my heart. I had a garage sale, and my grown daughter nearly flipped when she saw the rocking chair in the driveway with a price tag hanging from it. A twinge of guilt tugged at my heartstrings when she said, 'But that's the chair you used to rock me in when I was a baby.' I sheepishly took the chair back inside and told her it was hers now to keep.

"I tried to become a 'minimalist' and bought a shredder. I had six garage sales in four years and managed to make a few bucks in the process. Now when my friends come to the house, they ask, 'Where's all your stuff?' I laugh and tell them, 'Oh, there's still plenty. You haven't seen my closets!'"

Lauren suggests photographing your children's artwork as one space-saving strategy. Or make a "precious box" filled with only the items near and dear to your heart, such as report cards and handmade memorabilia. Then, pass it along to your grown children when the time is right.

Kathleen S., age 63, recalls her own mother's "mania" about purging. "When I was a child, my stuffed animals were my closest friends, and losing them suddenly all at once was devastatingly heartbreaking," Kathleen says. "I'd come home from playing outside to find my room stripped clean, my accumulated menagerie in the trash."

The moral of the purging story? If there are still family members living in (or visiting) the house, it's always a good idea to check with them first before whisking away their belongings to *Goodwill* or scheduling a pickup from the *Salvation Army*.

The Mind is a Terrible Thing to Lose

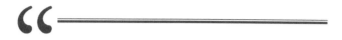

"The hubby and I spent half an hour backtracking at the outlet center looking for my lost car keys. Turned out I had them on me the entire time. Oops."

—Debbie H.

Menopausal women don't need another independent research study to tell us what we already know: We forget things. A lot. For anyone with a family history of Alzheimer's disease, a sudden onset of forgetfulness can be particularly alarming.

Because our reproductive systems tend to be similar to those of our own mothers, having a frank conversation about menopause might prove to be one more way to bond the mother-daughter relationship—provided your mom can recall that time of her life.

"It's not just walking into a room and not remembering why, but whole blocks of things (words, answers, details) usually found on the tips of our tongue [are] now gone," says Kathleen S. "It's like someone shook the Etch-a-Sketch. My mind is blank, when it didn't used to be."

Kathleen Shaputis believes many mothers of women in her generation, her own included, never told us about the quirks of menopause because they couldn't remember it themselves.

"We need to talk about this, especially with Alzheimer's being so prevalent today," Kathleen says. "It's not just the old cliché of walking into a room and forgetting why. It's so much more."

A frequent speaker at writers' conferences, Shaputis begins many workshops with an explanation of her tendency to get stuck in the middle of a sentence trying to find a word that was "right there a minute ago."

"The audience usually has a light chuckle. If the audience is primarily an older crowd, it's more like nods and smiles," Kathleen says.

Patricia N. has a theory about why some mothers don't approach the subject.

"I had a very open relationship with my mother," Patricia says. "She was frank and direct, a 'cool' mom. But somehow, this subject was just passed over, and I surmised that she probably just figured when it was my turn, I'd be shocked like hell, just like she was."

For women battling cancer and menopause, "chemo brain" and memory loss can be a double whammy.

Just the thought of getting behind the wheel of a car can be debilitating for some.

"I'm terrified of losing my memory while driving," Cindy W., age 58, says. "It feels like I'm losing my mind. The memory loss is like losing words that you used to know. They're right at the tip of the tongue but won't appear."

"I used to be good with people's names," says Carol G., age 67. "Now I use terms like 'hon' if I am not too close to a person, or 'darlin' if I am. Folks probably go away thinking, 'She is so sweet, bless her heart.'"

Beyond remembering names, double-checking to make sure the appliances are turned off is always a good idea. In menopause, it's a newfound ritual.

There's an Essential Oil for That!

Sprigs of rosemary have long been used as a symbol for remembrance. In Shakespeare's *Hamlet*, Ophelia says, "There's rosemary, that's for remembrance." (*Hamlet*, iv. 5.)

Today, rosemary essential oil has been gaining in popularity as an aid to enhance memory. Used as an aromatic or diffused, rosemary may improve memory and increase alertness.

Here's a funny story about menopause memory challenge.

A couple in their nineties are both having problems remembering things.

During a checkup, their doctor tells them that they're physically okay, but they might want to start writing things down to help them remember. Later that night, while watching TV, the old man gets up from his chair.

"Want anything while I'm in the kitchen?" he asks his wife.

"Will you get me a bowl of ice cream?" his wife answers.

"Sure."

"Don't you think you should write it down so you can remember it?" she asks.

"No, I can remember it."

"Well, I'd like some strawberries on top, too. Maybe you should write it down, so as not to forget it?"

"I can remember that. You want a bowl of ice cream with strawberries," he says.

"I'd also like whipped cream. I'm certain you'll forget that, write it down," she says.

"I don't need to write it down. I can remember it! Ice cream with strawberries and whipped cream. I got it, for goodness' sake!" he says, irritated.

The husband toddles into the kitchen. After about 20 minutes, the old man returns from the kitchen and hands his wife a plate of bacon and eggs. She stares at the plate for a moment.

"Where's my toast?" she asks.

Let's Get Organized!

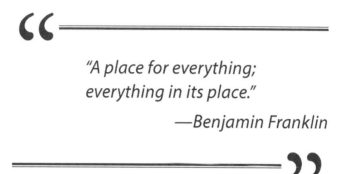

"A place for everything; everything in its place."

—*Benjamin Franklin*

Although memory loss might not be a symptom of menopause, but rather a typical symptom of aging in general, there are things we can all do to maximize our menopaused memory.

Interior designer *Linda Wallace*, owner of Divine Finds Interiors, provides her insight into how to organize your household, and how to avoid becoming a basket case when you lose things.

- Keep essentials visible and in the same place, every time. If you can see it, you'll remember where you put it, and you won't waste time and precious brain cells searching for your things.

- To avoid losing things, try to practice putting your keys, phone, glasses, and other valuables in the same place until it just becomes habit.

- Wear reading glasses? Don't even try to keep track of them. It's a waste of time. Because reading glasses can be found at the dollar store, simply buy them in bulk and keep them in practically every room in your house, including your garage, patio, and laundry room. (Who can read those tags?)

- Keep your essentials displayed attractively. You'll be more likely to keep things in the same place if you like the way these places look.

- Keys: Create drop-off locations at each main entry and exit to your home. Why two? Because, if you come in one way, the chances that you'll walk all the way to the other entrance without setting the keys down somewhere along the way are pretty slim. Avoid misplaced keys by keeping them only in these two locations. Use decorative bowls or baskets on entry tables or near back door entrances. It's much easier to drop than hang.

- Greeting cards: Off to a party, running late, and no birthday card? Think you bought one, but can't remember where you put it? Keep all greeting and thank-you cards in an antique tin box or a lidded basket. Make sure there's a pen in there, too (and maybe another pair of reading glasses).

Remember, just like in decorating, group "like items" together in one place.

- Rings: Place a small porcelain dish in up to three locations (depending on your habits): by the kitchen sink, near the bathroom lavatory, and next to your bed.

- Bracelets and necklaces: Consider interesting bowls for housing chunky jewelry and set them out on your vanity or dresser. Silver, porcelain, or wicker containers are as attractive as colorful flowers, but they require much less maintenance.

- Home office: Whether for appointments or invitations, bulletin boards are a must, and there is no shortage of attractive-looking ones found at stationery stores.

- Writing implements and miscellaneous: Display pens, pencils, and other office tools in a collection of decorative vases or ceramic pieces your child made in the first grade that you just can't throw away.

Organize before the lights go out.

- Night stand: Already in bed and don't feel like getting up? By your bed, in yet another pretty box, basket, or tray, keep your reading glasses, lip balm, hand lotion, a pen, and a small notepad for the "to-do list" you fret over in the middle of the night when you are undoubtedly wide awake.

"I write lists and use Post-it notes and check my calendar a hundred times a day and still forget where I'm supposed to be," says Jeri G., age 58.

Remember to remember!

Making "to-do lists" can help—as long as you remember where you put the list and try to remember that a.) you made a list, and b.) you need to look at the list.

Setting alarms on phones or clocks can also help, as long as they don't go ignored.

Susan M., age 56, always parks in the same spot.

"It just makes it easier to find the car," Susan says. "I don't like having to think of the easy, stupid things in life. I am a practical person. If you have routines, it makes it easier to multitask as some things become embedded as a standard process."

But making lists that are too long can also be overwhelming. Management coach Brendon Burchard, founder of www.ExpertsAcademy.com, shares his "list about making lists."

1. Keep a daily list and a master list.

2. Don't confuse lists with projects. A daily list contains single tasks (e.g., write a new resume). A master list contains projects or long-term tasks (e.g., learn Spanish).

3. To-do lists can be stressful. Make sure a list contains no more than 10 items and aim to cross off 5 each day.

4. If you feel a sense of achievement when you tick off the items on your list, you probably feel a sense of failure when you don't. Never add to a list without subtracting something from it.

5. By relying on lists, you limit your ability to experiment and try all the things that make life and work interesting. Lists should be a tool, not an obsession.

6. Never write down something on a list that you've already done for the pleasure of ticking it off. That way madness lies.

7. Bear in mind that if something is that important, you should remember it anyway. If it isn't so important, why write it down?

8. Don't make lists on the backs of envelopes. Keep your lists in one place, preferably on a smartphone linked to the cloud.

9. Boring speakers talk in lists: "And ninthly, let's examine collateral transformation swaps ..."

10. Don't round a list up to 10 if you don't need to.

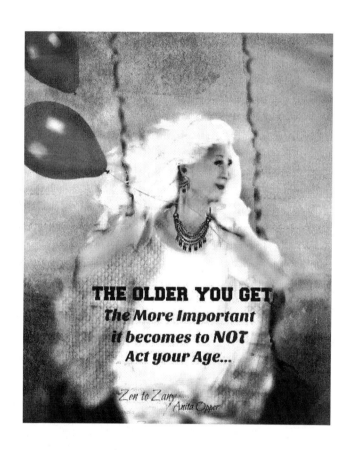

10

Is There a Light at the End of the Tunnel?

Is there such a thing as postmenopausal elation syndrome? Do things really go back to "normal"?

Roberta Perry, age 55, says yes.

"I can honestly tell you the day it all came back—my wits, my sense of womanhood, my balance, my sex drive," Roberta says. "Everything that had been a roller coaster for almost seven years finally came to a screeching halt—in a good way. I feel like myself again."

Roberta, the founder of *www.scrubzbody.com*, an all-natural skin care line, says following a healthy diet was her road to kick-starting balance and normalcy.

"Once I got nutritionally sound, everything seemed to be functioning properly," Roberta says. "I don't know how else to describe it; I just woke up feeling feminine again. I also notice that I have more tolerance now than when I was in menopause, as there were some months when I was so emotional, I never knew what to expect in terms of emotional mood swings and hot flashes. Don't wait for all those years of feeling crappy to catch up; I should have been taking better care of myself in general all along."

But is there really any truth to that sappy birthday card we've all seen: "Like fine wine, we improve with age"?

For Jan P., age 59, "life is good." The certified LEAP (lifestyle, eating, and performance) therapist also believes that eating well most of her life helped her to ease into postmenopause. "I think it's important to realize that symptoms hopefully are temporary." And while she's noticed some sagging skin, Jan has taken it in stride. "That's life. I don't need or want to remain looking 30 in my sixties."

Dr. Laura Berman believes "there is no such thing as a 'sexpiration' date anymore." The author of the *New York Times* bestseller *Real Sex for Real Women* has helped countless couples build stronger relationships, improve their sex lives, and achieve a heightened level of intimacy. Her latest book, *Quantum Love*, is all about using your body's atomic energy to create the relationships you desire. "You can't go back to the honeymoon phase, but there is something so much better within your reach," she promises.

Josephine R., 80-something, spends hours at the gym. In between her weight room, yoga, and water aerobics sessions, she's in the women's locker room, where she often chats with the other members in the sauna. It's not long before you learn about the passing of her husband of more than 50 years, and the fact that she no longer drives. Hang out with her long enough in the sauna and she'll tell you some other stories that will have you in tears and ashamed of the fact that you were just complaining about the pain you have in your left pinky. Her age-defying secrets, besides her obvious dedication to the weight room? "I eat healthy, keep active, and never stop fighting," pointing to her temple.

Of course, we can't turn back the clock, but we can control our future. In fact, menopause can be, and often is, liberating for many women. In many cases, it's a time for reinvention—as good a time as any to embark on a new career, relationship, or maybe both.

Entrepreneur and mixed media artist Anita Opper started a Facebook fan page called "Zen to Zany" in retirement. Opper, who describes her age as somewhere "between menopause and death, but I look more like I am in between PMS and hot flashes," says, "You never know what post menopause will bring to your life. Fast forward a few years, I have more than a million readers a week as well as an *Etsy* shop, and have made quite a bit of money, which is something I never expected."

Those blessed with their children's children are defying the stereotypical images of grandmothers, often welcoming any opportunity to explore their "inner child."

"I'm giving myself a break about the aging thing," says humorist *Vikki Claflin*, age 60, the bestselling author of *Chin Hairs & Back Fat*. "Middle age (and beyond) brings with it a certain peace. A letting go of the anxieties and often limited perspectives of youth. It's *liberating*.

"There's less drama. After six decades, we begin to realize that not *everything* is worth fighting over," Claflin adds. "As my grandma used to say, 'In 50 years, we'll all be dead and none of this will matter.'

"Learn to cherish your girlfriends," she continues. "We've attended Sally's four weddings, got Missy through three stints in rehab, and lived through Susie's douchy husband's affair. We've supported Jenny's new career as a nude art model, bailed Karen's son out of jail (again), and cried together when Linda got cancer. We have *history*.

"Discover new passions," Claflin says. "We're going back to school, learning new languages, traveling to new places, running marathons, and writing novels. We're not retiring. We're living longer than ever, and we're doing it in a red convertible. We laugh more. We see the silliness in things more easily. We're not as easily offended. Simply put, we've lightened up."

Age *is* just a number, and old rules no longer apply. Women are aging gracefully with style and ease. We are wearing our hair longer and aren't afraid of trends, whether it's a bold new shade of lipstick or taking up yoga for the first time. It may be the first time that some women actually are able to pay attention to themselves.

"Nothing matters anymore," says Paula R., age 61. "Your true friends are your true friends, your family is your family, and now you have to look at yourself and ask, 'What's my own legacy?' You've gained all kinds of knowledge, and now it's time to start focusing on the people around you whom you care about the most. I decided that I didn't want to leave this Earth before teaching my two daughters how to sew or how to plant flowers."

"Be brave and embrace new things," Paula adds. "You've already mastered what you can do. Now spend your time figuring out what you have never tried."

It's time to celebrate every paragraph and footnote in this crazy final chapter of womanhood. With every night sweat and sleepless night, isn't it about time we realized taking the time to love and cherish our new menopausal selves is the best way to spend the rest of our lives?

*"Do not regret growing older.
It's a privilege denied to many."*

—*Unknown*

ABOUT THE AUTHOR

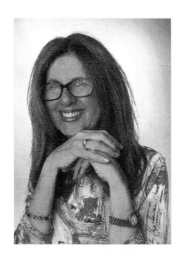

Linda Condrillo's debut book, *Period. The End,* was conceived right around the time of her first hot flash. Ten years, or approximately 10,000 night sweats later, and after countless intimate interviews with peri- and post-menopausal women and experts in the field, Linda is grateful to be able to share their wisdom, wit, and maybe a little whining to support women— many of whom might otherwise feel completely alone going through *The Change*.

A freelance writer since 2007, Linda has written feature articles for her local and online press. She currently writes human interest (and interesting humans) stories for her hometown news source, *TAPintoMountainside.net*.

Linda also shares "Everything you always wanted to know about frugality, but were afraid of sounding too cheap to ask," on her money-saving Facebook Fan Page, Frugalinda. Her penny-pinching tips have appeared in *Woman's Day Magazine, First for Women, CNNMoney.com, SpareFoot.com, TheStreet.com, GoBankingRates.com, and Wisebread.com.*

Besides writing, saving money, and writing about saving money, Linda enjoys aromatherapy, photography, and travel—especially to France. One of Linda's favorite pastimes is hanging out in cyberspace with like-minded Francophiles.

One year, unable to resist the urge to cross the pond, she took a solo trip to Paris to meet up with folks she met on travel message boards. Her children and husband warned her not to go—convinced she'd be kidnapped and left for dead in a bathtub full of ice cubes, sans one of her kidneys. She survived the trip (organs fully intact) and lived to write about the experience for *World Photo Adventure.com.*

Linda is the proud parent of two employed grown children, and is a new grandmother (best gig ever!). In addition to penning local stories in her spare time, Linda also sells real estate, and enjoys the good life in the suburbs of New Jersey with her retired husband.

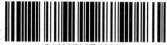

Made in the USA
San Bernardino, CA
29 October 2018